Innovations in Thoracic Surgery

Editor

KAZUHIRO YASUFUKU

THORACIC SURGERY CLINICS

www.thoracic.theclinics.com

Consulting Editor
M. BLAIR MARSHALL

May 2016 • Volume 26 • Number 2

ELSEVIER

1600 John F. Kennedy Boulevard • Suite 1800 • Philadelphia, Pennsylvania, 19103-2899

http://www.thoracic.theclinics.com

THORACIC SURGERY CLINICS Volume 26, Number 2
May 2016 ISSN 1547-4127, ISBN-13: 978-0-323-44481-1

Editor: John Vassallo (j.vassallo@elsevier.com)
Developmental Editor: Susan Showalter

Thoracic Surgery Clinics (ISSN 1547-4127) is published quarterly by Elsevier Inc., 360 Park Avenue South, New York, NY 10010-1710. Months of publication are February, May, August, and November. Business and editorial offices: 1600 John F. Kennedy Boulevard, Suite 1800, Philadelphia, PA 19103-2899. Periodicals postage paid at New York, NY, and additional mailing offices. Subscription prices are $355.00 per year (US individuals), $501.00 per year (US institutions), $100.00 per year (US Students), $435.00 per year (Canadian individuals), $648.00 per year (Canadian institutions), $225.00 per year (Canadian and international students), $465.00 per year (international individuals), and $648.00 per year (international institutions). Foreign air speed delivery is included in all Clinics' subscription prices. All prices are subject to change without notice. **POSTMASTER:** Send address changes to Thoracic Surgery Clinics, Elsevier Health Sciences Division, Subscription Customer Service, 3251 Riverport Lane, Maryland Heights, MO 63043. **Customer Service (orders, claims, online, change of address): Telephone: 1-800-654-2452 (U.S. and Canada); 314-447-8871 (outside U.S. and Canada). Fax: 314-447-8029. E-mail: journalscustomerservice-usa@elsevier.com (for print support); journalsonlinesupport-usa@elsevier.com (for online support).**

Reprints. For copies of 100 or more, of articles in this publication, please contact Commercial Rights Department, Elsevier Inc., 360 Park Avenue South, New York, NY 10010-1710. Tel: 212-633-3874; Fax: 212-633-3820; E-mail: reprints@elsevier.com.

Thoracic Surgery Clinics is covered in *MEDLINE/PubMed (Index Medicus), EMBASE/Excerpta Medica, Science Citation Index Expanded (SciSearch®), Journal Citation Reports/Science Edition,* and *Current Contents®/Clinical Medicine.*

Contributors

CONSULTING EDITOR

M. BLAIR MARSHALL, MD, FACS
Chief, Division of Thoracic Surgery;
Associate Professor, Department of Surgery,
Georgetown University Medical Center,
Georgetown University School of Medicine,
Washington, DC

EDITOR

KAZUHIRO YASUFUKU, MD, PhD
Director of Endoscopy, University Health
Network; Director, Interventional Thoracic
Surgery Program; Associate Professor,
Division of Thoracic Surgery, Toronto General
Hospital, University of Toronto, Toronto,
Ontario, Canada

AUTHORS

JONATHAN M. CHAREST, MS
Department of Surgery, Massachusetts
General Hospital, Boston, Massachusetts

YOLONDA L. COLSON, MD, PhD
Division of Thoracic Surgery, Department of
Surgery, Brigham and Women's Hospital;
Professor of Surgery, Division of Thoracic
Surgery, Brigham and Women's Hospital,
Harvard Medical School, Boston,
Massachusetts

MARCELO CYPEL, MD
Assistant Professor, Division of Thoracic
Surgery, Department of Surgery, Toronto
General Hospital, UHN, University of Toronto,
Toronto, Ontario, Canada

STEVEN R. DeMEESTER, MD
Professor and Clinical Scholar,
Department of Surgery, Keck School of
Medicine, The University of Southern
California, Los Angeles, California

CHRISTOPHER S. DIGESU, MD
Clinical Research Fellow, Division of
Thoracic Surgery, Department of Surgery,
Brigham and Women's Hospital, Boston,
Massachusetts

THOMAS R. GILDEA, MD, MS
Head, Section of Bronchology, Respiratory
Institute, Cleveland Clinic Foundation,
Cleveland, Ohio

SARAH E. GILPIN, PhD
Department of Surgery, Massachusetts
General Hospital, Harvard Medical School,
Boston, Massachusetts

DANIELA GOMPELMANN, MD
Member of the German Center for
Lung Research; Pneumology and
Critical Care Medicine, Thoraxklinik at
University of Heidelberg, Heidelberg,
Germany

DIEGO GONZALEZ-RIVAS, MD, FECTS
Minimally Invasive Thoracic Surgery Unit (UCTMI), Department of Thoracic Surgery, Coruña University Hospital, Coruña, Spain; Department of Thoracic Surgery, Shanghai Pulmonary Hospital, Tongji University School of Medicine, Shanghai, China

ERIC GOUDIE, MD
Research Fellow, Thoracic Surgery Laboratory, CHUM Endoscopic Tracheobronchial and Oesophageal Center (CETOC), Centre Hospitalier de l'Université de Montréal, Surgery Resident, University of Montreal, Montreal, Quebec, Canada

KEVIN L. GRIMES, MD
Assistant Professor, Department of Surgery, MetroHealth Medical Center, Cleveland, Ohio

MARK W. GRINSTAFF, PhD
Professor, Departments of Biomedical Engineering, Chemistry and Medicine, Metcalf Science Center, Boston University, Boston, Massachusetts

FELIX J.F. HERTH, PhD
Member of the German Center for Lung Research; Pneumology and Critical Care Medicine, Thoraxklinik at University of Heidelberg, Heidelberg, Germany

SOPHIE C. HOFFERBERTH, MBBS
General Surgery Resident, PGY2, Division of Thoracic Surgery, Department of Surgery, Brigham and Women's Hospital, Boston, Massachusetts

HARUHIRO INOUE, MD, PhD
Professor and Director, Digestive Disease Center, Showa University Koto-Toyosu Hospital, Tokyo, Japan

SATISH KALANJERI, MD, MRCP
Assistant Professor of Clinical Medicine, Interventional Pulmonology, Section of Pulmonary, Critical Care and Sleep Medicine, Louisiana State University Health Sciences Center, Shreveport, Louisiana

SHAF KESHAVJEE, MD
Professor of Surgery, Division of Thoracic Surgery, Department of Surgery, Toronto General Hospital, UHN, University of Toronto, Toronto, Ontario, Canada

BINIAM KIDANE, MD, MSc
Division of Thoracic Surgery, Toronto General Hospital, University Health Network, University of Toronto, Toronto, Ontario, Canada

MOISHE LIBERMAN, MD, PhD
Division of Thoracic Surgery, Associate Professor, Department of Surgery, Director, CHUM Endoscopic Tracheobronchial and Oesophageal Center (CETOC), Centre Hospitalier de l'Université de Montréal, University of Montreal, Montreal, Quebec, Canada

CALVIN NG, MD, FRCS
Division of Cardiothoracic Surgery, The Chinese University of Hong Kong, Prince of Wales Hospital, Hong Kong, China

HARALD C. OTT, MD
Department of Surgery, Massachusetts General Hospital, Harvard Medical School, Boston, Massachusetts

XI REN, PhD
Department of Surgery, Massachusetts General Hospital, Harvard Medical School, Boston, Massachusetts

MEHDI TAHIRI, MD
Research Fellow, Thoracic Surgery Laboratory, CHUM Endoscopic Tracheobronchial and Oesophageal Center (CETOC), Centre Hospitalier de l'Université de Montréal, Montreal, Quebec, Canada

STEPHANIE WORRELL, MD
Resident in Surgery, Department of Surgery, Keck School of Medicine, The University of Southern California, Los Angeles, California

YANG YANG, MD
Department of Thoracic Surgery, Shanghai Pulmonary Hospital, Tongji University School of Medicine, Shanghai, China

KAZUHIRO YASUFUKU, MD, PhD
Director of Endoscopy, University Health Network; Director, Interventional Thoracic Surgery Program; Associate Professor, Division of Thoracic Surgery, Toronto General Hospital, University of Toronto, Toronto, Ontario, Canada

Contents

Different modalities of surgical excisional biopsy can be used when needle biopsy fails to provide tissue diagnosis. These modalities include intraoperative localization techniques, such as ultrasonography, and preoperative localization techniques, such as liquid dyes, radiolabeled aggregates, hook wires, microcoils, and navigational bronchoscopy techniques. The highest level of evidence for efficacy currently appears to support microcoils, radiolabeling, and hook-wire localization techniques. Multiple methods have been used to help identify intersegmental planes to facilitate minimally invasive segmental resection. These methods include use of 3-dimensional multidetector computed tomographic rendering, administration of dyes such as indocyanine green, and virtual bronchoscopic techniques.

Isolated lung perfusion (ILP) has been examined and developed in lung transplantation and thoracic oncology research. In lung transplantation, ILP has been used to assess physiologic integrity of donor lungs after removal from the donor, and it has also been proposed as a method for active treatment and repair of injured unsuitable donor organs ex vivo. ILP is attractive as a concept to deliver high-dose chemotherapy to treat pulmonary metastatic disease, referred to as in vivo lung perfusion. This article focuses on the rationale, technical aspects, and experimental and clinical experience of in vivo lung perfusion. A perspective on the future application of these techniques are described.

Historically, the most robust outcomes in treatment of achalasia were seen with surgical myotomy. Per oral endoscopic myotomy (POEM) introduced an endoscopic method for creating a surgical myotomy. Thousands of cases of POEM have been performed; however, there is no standard technique, and the rates of clinical success and adverse events vary widely among centers. This article presents a detailed description of the POEM technique, including the rationale and potential pitfalls of the main variations, in the context of the international literature.

Whole lung extracellular matrix scaffolds can be created by perfusion of cadaveric organs with decellularizing detergents, providing a platform for organ regeneration. Lung epithelial engineering must address both the proximal airway cells that function to metabolize toxins and aid mucociliary clearance and the distal pneumocytes that facilitate gas exchange. Engineered pulmonary vasculature must support in vivo blood perfusion with low resistance and intact barrier function and be antithrombotic. Repopulating the native lung matrix with sufficient cell numbers in appropriate anatomic locations is required to enable organ function.

Endoscopic resection and ablation have become the preferred therapy for most patients with high-grade dysplasia or superficial esophageal cancer. Endoscopic therapy offers esophageal preservation with similar oncologic outcomes and significantly fewer complications compared with the alternative of esopahgectomy. The goal of endotherapy is eradication of all the premalignant intestinal metaplasia to minimize the risk for metachronous cancer development. Once accomplished, careful follow-up is necessary to address recurrent intestinal metaplasia or dysplasia and prevent long-term failure of an endoscopic approach in these patients.

Endoscopic lung volume reduction (ELVR) presents an effective therapy in patients with advanced emphysema. Different ELVR techniques are available differing in mechanism of action, degree of reversibility and safety. Precise patient selection with respect to pulmonary function test, emphysema distribution, and collateral ventilation are prerequisites for a successful use of the various ELVR techniques. To date, there are only a few randomized controlled trials for bronchoscopic therapy in patients with chronic obstructive pulmonary disease, so the various techniques should be performed within clinical trials or registry studies.

 Video content accompanies this article at http://www.thoracic.theclinics.com

Uniportal video-assisted thoracic surgery (VATS) represents a radical change in the approach to lung resection compared with conventional VATS. Because the placement of the surgical instruments and the camera is done through the same incision, uniportal VATS can pose a challenge for both the surgeon and the assistant. Recent industry improvements have made single-port VATS easier to learn. We can expect more developments of subcostal or embryonic natural orifice translumenal endoscopic surgery access, improvements in 3D image systems, single-port robotics, and wireless cameras. The advances in digital technology may facilitate the adoption of the uniportal VATS technique.

Electromagnetic navigational bronchoscopy is a useful addition to the array of modalities available to sample peripheral lung lesions. Its utility in diagnosing peripheral lesions has been steadily increasing since the Food and Drug Administration first approved it in 2004. The improvement can be attributed to continuous refinement in technology, increasing training and experience with the procedure, perhaps widespread availability of rapid onsite cytologic evaluation, and better patient selection. It may also be attributable to improvements of the technology and more available tools to perform biopsy of the peripheral lung.

Nanotechnology is an emerging field with potential as an adjunct to cancer therapy, particularly thoracic surgery. Therapy can be delivered to tumors in a more targeted fashion, with less systemic toxicity. Nanoparticles may aid in diagnosis, preoperative characterization, and intraoperative localization of thoracic tumors and their lymphatics. Focused research into nanotechnology's ability to deliver both diagnostics and therapeutics has led to the development of nanotheranostics, which promises to improve the treatment of thoracic malignancies through enhanced tumor targeting, controlled drug delivery, and therapeutic monitoring. This article reviews nanoplatforms, their unique properties, and the potential for clinical application in thoracic surgery.

In the last decade, many energy devices have entered day-to-day practice in thoracic surgery. Some have proven and recognized applications, whereas others still require further trials. Nevertheless, currently used devices continue to be improved on and new applications for current devices will be evaluated. Ultimately, novel applications of energy in thoracic surgery and refinement in technology will hopefully allow for safer and less invasive techniques for patients requiring thoracic surgical procedures. In this article, we review the present and future applications of energy devices in thoracic surgery.

THORACIC SURGERY CLINICS

THE CLINICS ARE AVAILABLE ONLINE!
Access your subscription at:
www.theclinics.com

Errata

In the February 2016 issue (Volume 26, Number 1), the synopsis for the article "Is Surgery Warranted for Oligometastatic Disease?" by Tom Treasure and Fergus Macbeth is different than that which the authors intended. The correct synopsis for the article is as follows:

Removing or ablating pulmonary metastases is an increasingly common procedure especially when they are the first or only site of relapse. This is assumed to benefit the patients and lead to health gain including prolonged survival. The authors are unaware of any studies confirming or quantifying clinical benefit. This article strongly challenges the belief in the overall effectiveness of metastasectomy and shows that it is not supported by a sound biological rationale or any good evidence. Reasons are suggested why this unfounded belief has become so prevalent.

In the February 2016 issue (Volume 26, Number 1), in the article "Results of Pulmonary Resection" by Karen J. Dickinson and Shanda H. Blackmon, the credit line for Table 1 was erroneously omitted. Table 1, "Summary of survival outcomes and prognostic factors in recently published studies," should have been accompanied by the following credit line:

From Kim HK, Cho JH, Lee HY, et al. Pulmonary metastasectomy for colorectal cancer: How many nodules, how many times? WJG 2014;20:6133–45.

The authors apologize for failing to credit the original source for Table 1.

Thorac Surg Clin 26 (2016) ix
http://dx.doi.org/10.1016/j.thorsurg.2016.02.002
1547-4127/16/$ – see front matter © 2016 Elsevier Inc. All rights reserved.

Preface
Innovations in Thoracic Surgery

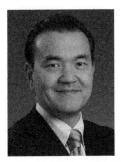

Kazuhiro Yasufuku, MD, PhD
Editor

Since the first successful one-stage pneumonectomy for lung cancer performed by Dr Evarts Graham in 1933, modern thoracic surgery has evolved significantly. Various technology introduced over time has advanced thoracic surgery from open procedures to minimally invasive surgeries. Perhaps one of the most significant developments in thoracic surgery has been the advent of video-assisted thoracoscopic surgery (VATS). The invention of the Charged Coupled Device Image Sensor has allowed miniaturization of surgical cameras, thus allowing the use of the high-definition thoracoscope during minimally invasive surgeries. New developments in surgical instruments, stapling devices, and energy devices have allowed surgeons to perform more advanced and complex VATS procedures. Surgical robotic technology has also emerged as an approach to a different dimension of minimally invasive surgery.

Development of technology in endoscopy has set a new standard for ultraminimally invasive thoracic procedures. Now, incisionless endoscopic surgeries can be performed for benign esophageal disease and to manage patients with early-stage esophageal cancer. Novel bronchoscopic technologies, including navigational bronchoscopy and endobronchial ultrasound, have opened up alternatives to invasive diagnostic/therapeutic procedures for lung cancer. There are various types of technology that have been developed for bronchoscopic lung volume reduction for the management of patients with chronic obstructive pulmonary disease. Endoscopic/bronchoscopic procedures are now being utilized in combination with advanced imaging during VATS for management of thoracic malignancies.

In this issue of *Thoracic Surgery Clinics*, innovations in thoracic procedures are reviewed with contributions from the experts in the field. The different technical aspects of new technologies currently available for thoracic surgeons are discussed. In addition, new technologies on the horizon, including nanotechnology, isolated lung perfusion technology, and bioengineered organs, are introduced. I would like to thank all of the contributing authors for their expertise and contributions to this issue.

Kazuhiro Yasufuku, MD, PhD
University Health Network
Interventional Thoracic Surgery Program
Division of Thoracic Surgery
Toronto General Hospital
University of Toronto
200 Elizabeth Street, 9N-957
Toronto, ON M5K 2C4, Canada

E-mail address:
kazuhiro.yasufuku@uhn.ca

Thorac Surg Clin 26 (2016) xi
http://dx.doi.org/10.1016/j.thorsurg.2016.02.001
1547-4127/16/$ – see front matter © 2016 Published by Elsevier Inc.

Advances in Image-Guided Thoracic Surgery

Biniam Kidane, MD, MSc, Kazuhiro Yasufuku, MD, PhD*

KEYWORDS

- Non-small-cell lung carcinoma • Pulmonary surgical procedures
- Minimally invasive surgical procedures • Neoplasm invasiveness

KEY POINTS

- Different modalities of surgical excisional biopsy can be used when needle biopsy has failed to provide tissue diagnosis.
- These modalities include intraoperative localization techniques, such as ultrasonography, and preoperative localization techniques, such as liquid dyes, radiolabeled aggregates, hook wires, and microcoils, as well as navigational bronchoscopy techniques.
- The highest level of evidence for efficacy currently appears to support microcoils, radiolabeling, and hook-wire localization techniques.
- Multiple methods have been used to help identify intersegmental planes in order to facilitate minimally invasive segmental resection.
- These methods include use of 3-dimensional multidetector computed tomographic rendering, administration of dyes such as indocyanine green, and virtual bronchoscopic techniques.

INTRODUCTION

There has been increasing use of imaging technology to facilitate minimally invasive thoracic surgery techniques. This article reviews the use of imaging technology to facilitate minimally invasive excisional biopsy of small pulmonary nodules as well as the use of imaging technology to facilitate minimally invasive segmental lung resection.

LOCALIZATION OF SMALL PULMONARY NODULES

Increasing use of low-dose computed tomographic (CT) screening for lung cancer has resulted in increased detection of small peripheral nodules or semisolid ground-glass opacities (GGOs). Although many of these may be amenable to percutaneous, image-guided needle biopsy, these lesions are challenging because of their small size and risk of sampling error with needle biopsy. Semisolid GGOs are even more challenging given their semisolid state. Different modalities of surgical excisional biopsy have been used to address these challenges when needle biopsy has failed to provide tissue diagnosis.

Video-assisted thoracoscopic surgery (VATS) or open biopsy directed by intraoperative finger palpation or instrument sliding technique has been reported to have localization rates of approximately 30%.[1] The following is a review of image-guided pulmonary nodule localization.

Intraoperative Localization with Ultrasonography

Use of intraoperative ultrasonography has been reported to yield localization rates of up to 93%.[1–3] In their prospective nonrandomized study, Khereba and colleagues[1] found that

Conflicts of Interest: None to declare.
Division of Thoracic Surgery, Toronto General Hospital, University Health Network, University of Toronto, 200 Elizabeth Street, 9N-957, Toronto M5G 2C4, Ontario, Canada
* Corresponding author.
E-mail address: kazuhiro.yasufuku@uhn.ca

Thorac Surg Clin 26 (2016) 129–138
http://dx.doi.org/10.1016/j.thorsurg.2015.12.001
1547-4127/16/$ – see front matter © 2016 Elsevier Inc. All rights reserved.

intraoperative ultrasonography localized an additional 43% (n = 20/46) of nodules that were not identified by palpation or visualization. Furthermore, intraoperative ultrasonography is not associated with complications related to its use. However, deflation of the lung is mandatory for visualization of the nodule, and therefore, its use in patients with emphysema is more challenging.[2,3] Moreover, ultrasonography is highly operator-dependent. Khereba and colleagues[1] reported mean operative times of 74 +/− 34 minutes.[1] They also found however that the learning curve was quite steep and that the time required to identify a nodule sonographically decreased to an average of 4 minutes after the first few cases. The steepness of the learning curve is highlighted by the fact that 3 of 4 surgeons performing these procedures had no formal ultrasound training before the study.[1] The ultrasound probes that were used in these studies were mainly made for application in the abdominal cavity; thus, the settings may not be ideal for use in the lung. Currently, new thoracoscopic ultrasound probes are in development, which may enhance the localization capabilities within the lung.[4]

Preoperative Percutaneous Insertion of Hook Wire and Suture

The hook-wire and suture technique involves preoperative insertion of a short 1-cm hook with an attached 30-cm monofilament suture that is exteriorized on the skin (**Fig. 1**).[5] Insertion is accomplished under CT guidance on the same day as VATS excisional biopsy.[5] Use of hook-wire localization has been reported to yield localization rates of up to 94% in retrospective studies.[5] Approximately 2% to 4% of patients experienced postinsertion pneumothoraces that required placement of chest tubes before proceeding to excisional biopsy.[5,6] Although a significant limitation reported

independently is a high rate of hook-wire dislodgement of up to 10%, recent data from the group that pioneered the hook-wire approach suggest that there is a low (1%–2%) rate of dislodgement of the hook wire between insertion and excisional biopsy.[5,7,8] A rare complication that has been reported is massive air embolism; it has mainly been described in case reports and 1 large case series at a rate of 0.6% (n = 1/161).[9] Furthermore, Miyoshi and colleagues[5] suggest that this risk can be mitigated by limiting the length of time required to insert the hook-wire system.

Preoperative Percutaneous Injection of Radiolabeled Aggregates

Preoperative injection of radiolabeled aggregates under CT guidance has been used to successfully localize nodules. Galetta and colleagues[10] reported a series of 123 nodules in 112 patients that they preoperatively localized using Technitium-99 radiolabeled macroaggregates. Intraoperatively, they used a handheld gamma probe to detect the area to resect.[10] Mean nodule size was 9 mm (with a range of 3–24 mm), and mean distance from the pleura was 12 mm (with a range of 0–39 mm).[10] They reported 62.5% (n = 30/44) successful VATS biopsy with the rest requiring biopsy via thoracotomy. The gamma probe failed to localize the nodule entirely (either by VATS or thoracotomy) in only 2 patients (1.8%).[10] In terms of complications, they reported 29.4% (n = 33) asymptomatic pneumothoraces with only 1 patient requiring chest tube insertion and 2 cases (1.8%) of significant radiotracer extravasation into the pleural cavity.[10]

A randomized controlled trial (RCT) comparing hook-wire localization to radio-guided localization in small 6- to 19-mm nodules showed that there was not a statistically significant difference between the 2 modalities with localization rates of

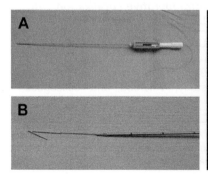
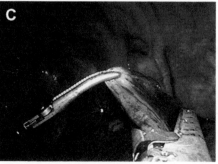

Fig. 1. Hook-wire localization. (*A*) Hook-wire device used for localization. (*B*) Hook wire with the suture deployed from the device. (*C*) Intraoperative findings of VATS wedge resection of a lung nodule with hook-wire localization.

84% (n = 21/25) and 96% (n = 24/25), respectively.[11] Finger palpation was also attempted in both arms of the study and resulted in 24% and 28% localization rates in each arm, respectively; both modalities were significantly better at localizing the nodule than finger palpation.[11] Complications were limited to pneumothoraces in 24% and 4% of patients, respectively; however, these did not require any additional chest drainage.[11]

Preoperative Percutaneous Insertion of Microcoils

Preoperative CT-guided percutaneous insertion of microcoils has been successfully used to achieve fluoroscopy-guided resection intraoperatively. Hajjar and colleagues[12] reported the use of this technique in a prospective series of 74 patients with deep lung nodules (less 2 cm in size) after a history of previous malignancy. They reported successful microcoil insertion in all patients with only 2 (2.7%) microcoil displacements at time of lung isolation.[12] They reported no complications other than a 4% (n = 3) asymptomatic pneumothorax rate, which required no interventions.[12] With a mean operative time of 52.5 ± 24.5 minutes, they reported 100% successful VATS excision with no need to convert to thoracotomy.[12]

More recently, Finley and colleagues[13] reported the results of a randomized trial supporting the use of microcoils in patients with nodules smaller than 15 mm. In the experimental group, platinum microcoils were inserted preoperatively under CT guidance, and these were then identified intraoperatively via fluoroscopy (**Fig. 2**).[13] In the control group, intraoperative localization was accomplished using visual inspection and finger palpation.[13] The use of microcoils resulted in significantly higher localization rates with 93% (n = 27/29) achieving diagnosis with VATS excision alone compared with the finger palpation group, which had a localization rate of 48% (n = 13/27).[13] Although the microcoil group required the use of preoperative radiologic localization and intraoperative fluoroscopy, there was no significant difference in cost between the 2 groups.[13] The lack of significant difference was likely due to the fact that higher costs associated with preoperative microcoil insertion were offset by significantly decreased operative time (37 ± 39 vs 100 ± 67 minutes; P<.001) and decreased stapler firings in the microcoil group.[13] Although there was a 13% pneumothorax rate in the microcoil group, none of these required chest tube drainage.[13] Kha and colleagues[14] recently reported a modification of this technique wherein the entire microcoil is inserted in the lung rather than

Finley's method, wherein part of the coil is left on the surface of the lung. Kha and colleagues[14] compared these 2 methods in 63 patients and found that the modified technique resulted in decreased CT procedure time and radiation dose, while not being associated with any reductions in complete resection rates or increases in complications.

A recent study prospectively compared outcomes between inserting microcoils through the lesion versus adjacent to the lesion and found that there were no significant differences in localization or complication rates.[15] Although described as a randomized study, it is not clear whether this was truly randomized. Nevertheless, the results in 101 patients show similar safety and efficacy.[15]

Preoperative Percutaneous Injection of Liquid Agents

Alternative techniques to preoperatively localize nodules include injection of liquid/contrast agents such as methylene blue dye, India ink, iodine, barium, cyanoacrylate, or lipiodol.[16–22]

Although shown to be successful, use of methylene blue alone has been associated with 13% failure rate in localization.[11,23] Furthermore, because of rapid diffusion of the dye, excision must be completed within 3 hours of methylene blue injection or risk further increases in failure rate.[23] Preoperative injection of lipiodol is not subject to such time sensitivity because it can last for 3 months, and thus, its use does not require the coordination of operating room and radiology department resources.[21] Watanabe and colleagues[21] reported 100% localization rates in their retrospective study of 174 nodules but also reported a 17% (n = 30) rate of pneumothorax, with only 6% (n = 11) requiring a chest tube. They also reported that 1 person required emergency thoracotomy for hemopneumothorax.[21] These nodules had a mean size of 10 ± 6 mm (range of 2–30 mm) and had a mean distance from the pleura of 10 ± 7 mm (range of 0–30 mm).[21] In a more recent series of lipiodol use, Mogi and colleagues[22] reported 100% successful localization and VATS excision in 56 patients. Lipiodol can either be used alone and visualized intraoperatively by fluoroscopy or be paired with a colored collagen obviating fluoroscopy. Watanabe and colleagues[21] initially used the latter technique but then switched to the fluoroscopy technique because of the high cost of using collagen.

Navigational Bronchoscopy Techniques

An even less-invasive approach to preoperative localization is the use of navigational bronchoscopy

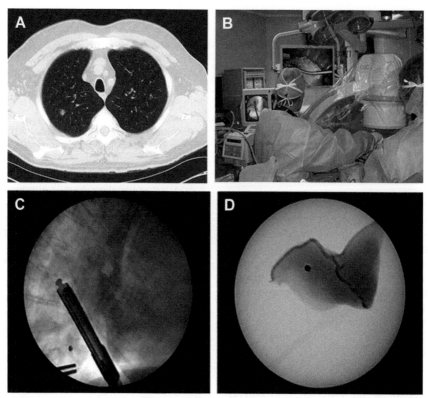

Fig. 2. Microcoil localization. (*A*) Preoperative CT scan showing a subcentimeter GGO in the right upper lobe. (*B*) Fluoroscopy-guided VATS wedge resection in a regular operating room. (*C*) Fluoroscopy images of the endostapler and the microcoil. (*D*) Fluoroscopy used to confirm the microcoil within the resected specimen.

techniques to mark a nodule or implant a fiducial for targeting an excisional biopsy. Electromagnetic navigational bronchoscopy uses sensor-location technology in concert with a 3-dimensional (3D) reconstruction of CT scan data in order to guide a bronchoscopic probe to a lung nodule[24,25]; this yields a virtual bronchoscopic reconstruction that can be paired with true bronchoscopic images to facilitate injection of dye or fiducial.

Krimsky and colleagues[24] reported an 81% detection rate (n = 17/21) of nodules with a mean size of 13.4 mm using injection of indigo carmine or methylene blue dye via electromagnetic navigational bronchoscopy followed by VATS or robotic wedge resection. Bolton and colleagues[25] reported 100% localization in 11 patients using methylene blue dye via electromagnetic navigational bronchoscopy followed by robotic wedge resection. Both studies reported no need for conversion to open resection or adverse events related to the marking procedure.[24,25]

Asano and colleagues[26] used a similar technique using virtual navigational bronchoscopy with barium sulfate suspension and localized the lesion intraoperatively with fluoroscopy-assisted VATS. They reported 100% detection rate in 23 patients with no conversion to thoracotomy and no complications.[26] Median nodule size was 7 mm (range of 5–10 mm) and median distance from pleura was 7 mm (range of 1–20 mm).[26]

Miyoshi and colleagues[27] reported a 100% detection rate with only 1 (11.1%) conversion to mini-thoracotomy in an early series of 9 patients that underwent virtual navigational bronchoscopy-guided insertion of a microcoil. Mean nodule size was 11 mm (range of 5–17 mm), and mean distance from pleura was 9 mm (range of 0–15 mm).[27] The mean time between marking and VATS was 7 days, and no complications were reported.[27]

Summary

Thus, there are multiple modalities to localize small pulmonary nodules that have improved on visual inspection and finger palpation (**Table 1**). Although there are promising data for intraoperative ultrasonography, there is neither RCT evidence nor any prospective studies comparing ultrasonography to modalities other than palpation. It is also not being used in many centers. Some promising data exist for the use of navigational bronchoscopy as a means to localize

Table 1
Review of localization techniques

Technique	Advantages	Disadvantages
Palpation (finger or instrument)	No additional equipment cost	50%–70% failure rate
Percutaneous techniques		
Microcoils	Up to 100% success Good randomized evidence Equivalent cost to palpation	Up to 13% pneumothorax, rarely need chest tube 2.7% microcoil displacement —
Hook wire	Up to 94% success Randomized evidence —	Up to 24% pneumothorax rate 2%–4% pneumothoraces requiring chest tubes 2%–10% hook-wire dislodgement Rare risk of air embolism
Radiolabeled aggregates	Up to 96% success Randomized evidence	4%–29% pneumothorax, rarely need chest tube Nuclear medicine coordination
Methylene blue injection	Low cost —	High failure rate (up to 13%) Requires wedge resection within 3 h Dye diffusion between injection and resection No information on depth
Lipiodol injection	Up to 100% success Can last for months	Up to 17% pneumothorax rate 6% pneumothoraces requiring chest tubes No information on depth Potential risks of embolism Few case series
Intraoperative ultrasound	Up to 93% success No complications	Requires lung deflation Highly operator-dependent Unreliable in emphysematous lung Limited data on reproducibility
Navigational bronchoscopic techniques	Up to 100% success rate No complications	Few case series Cost

nodules for resection; however, further human evidence is needed. The highest level of evidence for efficacy currently appears to support microcoils, radiolabeling, and hook-wire localization techniques.[11,13] However, these randomized trials have important limitations to keep in mind. The radiolabeling-versus-hook-wire trial was likely underpowered to detect a difference between those 2 modalities, and the microcoil trial only focused on a comparison against finger palpation rather than comparing against a modality known to be more effective (eg, radiolabeling, hook wire, dye, etc.).[11,13] A best evidence review published in 2012 suggested that radiolabeling may be preferable; however, that review did not take into consideration the growing recent literature on microcoils and hook-wire techniques.[28]

At the authors' institution, we predominantly use microcoils. We also have imaging capabilities in specially-built guided therapeutic operating room, which includes a robotic cone-beam CT and a dual-source CT scanner, that allow to perform image-guided interventions

intraoperatively without the need for transport[29] (**Fig. 3**). These capabilities may have implications in terms of time- and cost-savings as well as reduction in rate of dislodgements, which are of serious concern especially in hook-wire localization. Furthermore, centralization of the procedure entirely inside the operating room removes the worry about pneumothoraces after the marking procedure.

IMAGE GUIDANCE FOR SEGMENTAL RESECTION
Three-Dimensional Multidetector Computed Tomographic Rendering

Multiple groups have described the use of rendered images from 3D multidetector CT angiography to create a 3D map to guide segmentectomy (**Table 2**).[30–35]

Oizumi and colleagues[30–32] used this method, which they termed SAMURAI (Segmentectomy Achieved by MDCT for Use in Respective Anatomic Interpretation), and described the use

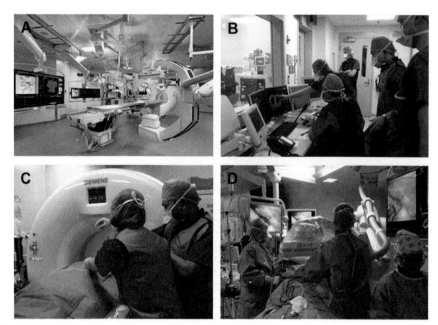

Fig. 3. Guided therapeutic operating room. (*A*) The 1200-square-feet operating room at the Toronto General Hospital houses the state-of-the-art imaging equipment, including the robotic cone-beam CT and the dual source-dual energy CT scanner and high-end endoscopic technology capable of minimally invasive image-guided surgery. (*B*) Image planning in the control room during CT-guided intervention. (*C*) CT-guided microcoil insertion performed in the guided therapeutic operating room immediately before VATS resection. (*D*) VATS wedge resection with image guidance using intraoperative cone-beam CT.

Table 2
Review of image-guided segmental resection techniques

Technique	Description	Outcomes
3D multidetector CT	Multislice CT angiography, then volume rendering and 3D reconstruction	• 98%–100% successful VATS segmental resections • No specific complications related to image guidance
Virtual-assisted lung mapping	Virtual bronchoscopy to select appropriate bronchial branches then injection of indigo carmine	• 98%–100% successful VATS segmental resections • Up to 4% rate of pneumothorax after marking, none requiring chest drainage
Dye-based identification of intersegmental planes		
Transbronchial administration	Transbronchial administration of ICG after clamping of target bronchus, then visualization of intersegmental planes via infrared scope	• 100% successful VATS segmental resections • No specific complications related to image-guidance • ICG lasts longer than when administered intravenously
Intravenous administration	Intravenous administration of ICG after transection of target pulmonary vasculature, then visualization of intersegmental planes via infrared scope	• 100% successful identification and segmental resections • No specific complications related to image guidance • Short period of ICG staining

of multislice CT angiography with segmentation and color coding of arteries and veins. These images are then volume-rendered, and 3D images are produced. These images can then be manipulated as necessary during surgery (ie, magnification, rotation).[30–32] The parenchymal resection margins were identified through the visualization of the inflation-deflation line after ligation of the bronchus and inflation of the lung (ie, clamp and inflate).[30–32] Oizumi and colleagues[31] reported this method in a series of 52 patients undergoing VATS segmentectomy. They reported a 98% (n = 51/52) VATS segmentectomy rate with only 1 patient requiring conversion to thoracotomy for control of pulmonary arterial bleeding.[31] There were no mortalities or local recurrences reported.[31] In a recent review article, Oizumi and colleagues[32] informally updated these results and reported that they have now performed 160 cases with 98% VATS success rate and 100% 5-year overall survival rate after a mean follow-up of 3.5 years.

Iwano and colleagues[35] described the use of similar imaging methods to also model and superimpose a spherical virtual surgical safety margin around the tumor. Using this method, they reported a series of 17 tumors (≤2 cm in diameter) in 16 patients who had no positive margins in their segmentectomy specimens.

Kanzaki and colleagues[33] reported a series of 57 patients with stage IA lung cancer on whom VATS segmentectomies were planned using these 3D CT methods. They reported 100% success rate in completion of VATS segmentectomies with mean operative times of 187 ± 47 minutes. There were no intraoperative complications and few postoperative complications with the most common being prolonged air leak (>6 days) in 10 patients (17.5%).[33] With a mean follow-up duration of 2.6 ± 1.3 years, they reported a 5-year overall survival rate of 88.6% and local recurrence in 8.8% of patients (n = 5).[33]

These methods may be further enhanced or aided through the use of 3D printing, which would allow surgeons to physically hold and manipulate the 3D model in their hands.[36]

Dye-Based Methods

Indocyanine green (ICG) has been used extensively to help identify intersegmental planes in order to facilitate segmental resection. Other dyes have also been used such as methylene blue.[37]

Oh and colleagues[38] described a method of first ligating the segmental veins and arteries and then injecting ICG through the ligated segmental bronchus. They report that this allows for change of color in the parenchyma and surface of the segment to be resected.[38] This technique did not require any specialized imaging modalities other than VATS.

Sekine and colleagues[39] described a method of transbronchial instillation of ICG and then using an infrared-based ICG fluorescence endoscope to help visualize the ICG fluorescence and thus the intersegmental planes. They reported their results in 10 patients using this method as compared with 10 matched patients who underwent segmental resections using traditional "clamp-and-inflate" methods.[39] They reported no significant differences between groups in terms of operative time, blood loss, or complications.[39] Sekine and colleagues[39] noted that the limitation of intravascular administration of ICG is that it does not last as long if administered transbronchially.

Misaki and colleagues[40] described 8 patients in whom they used intravenous administration of ICG after segmental pulmonary artery ligation.[40] Infrared thoracoscopy was used to visualize the intersegmental plane, and this appeared as a "white-to-blue" transition zone. On average, staining appeared within 13 seconds, reached maximal staining at about 28 seconds after administration, and lasted for about 210 seconds.[40]

Use of intravenous administration of ICG after segmental pulmonary vascular ligation has also been described during robotic segmentectomy[41] and has been mainly using a 1-wavelength platform.[41] In general, ICG detection via infrared thoracoscopy is by either 2-wavelength or 1-wavelength platforms.[42] The 2-wavelength platforms detect absorption at 2 wavelengths and produce an image of the difference between those 2 wavelengths; thus, ICG-rich areas show up as a blue color, whereas ICG-deficient areas show up as white.[42] The 1-wavelength platform detects absorption at 1 wavelength and produces a fluorescent image for ICG-rich areas.[42] Kasai and colleagues[42] reported a series of 30 patients in whom they compared these methods; in this study, they used the 2-wavelength platform in 10 patients, whereas they used the 1-wavelength platform in 20 patients. ICG was administered via a peripheral vein after ligation of segmental arteries, veins, and bronchi.[42] The borders for resection were well-demarcated in 90% and 95% for 2-wavelength or 1-wavelength platforms, respectively.[42] The staining duration was significantly longer in the 1-wavelength platform (median 370 seconds with interquartile range of 296–440 vs median 220 seconds with interquartile range of 187–251).[42] Furthermore, the 1-wavelength platform required lower ICG doses.[42] Thus, this suggested that 1-wavelength platforms may be preferable.[42]

Virtual-Assisted Lung Mapping

Virtual-assisted lung mapping combines virtual bronchoscopic techniques, 3D CT rendering, and dye-based techniques to facilitate minimally invasive segmentectomy.[43–45]

Sato and colleagues[43–45] described the use of virtual bronchoscopy under local anesthesia to select several appropriate bronchial branches for marking.[43–45] The location of the catheter tip for marking was confirmed by fluoroscopy and followed by injection of indigo carmine. Afterward, 3D multidetector CT was used to produce 3D virtual images to be used intraoperatively to facilitate resection.[43–45] They described the use of this method in wedge resection or segmentectomy of hardly palpable lung tumors/nodules.[43–45] For wedge resections, they used 2 to 3 markings in order to surround the tumor and thus delineate the zone of resection.[44] For segmentectomies, they used 3 to 6 markings to delineate the intersegmental planes for resection.[44] They reported a series of 70 lung tumors that were resected via 63 segmentectomies using this method.[44] They reported that 69 of 70 (98.5%) lesions had successful resection with good resection margins with only 1 requiring step-up to lobectomy due to inadequate margins.[44] In this single-center study, surgeons rated the VAL-MAP technique to be most helpful for wedge resections or complex segmentectomies of small, hardly palpable tumors.[44] Average bronchoscopy time was 20.1 ± 5.65 minutes.[44] Markings were made within 2 days of the surgery.[44] No major complications were reported. The investigators described 4 minor pneumothoraces that were identified in the CT scans after the marking procedure; these minor pneumothoraces were asymptomatic and did not require treatment.[44]

REFERENCES

1. Khereba M, Ferraro P, Duranceau A, et al. Thoracoscopic localization of intraparenchymal pulmonary nodules using direct intracavitary thoracoscopic ultrasonography prevents conversion of VATS procedures to thoracotomy in selected patients. J Thorac Cardiovasc Surg 2012;144:1160–5.

2. Mattioli S, D'Ovidio F, Daddi N, et al. Transthoracic endosonography for the intraoperative localization of lung nodules. Ann Thorac Surg 2005;79:443–9 [discussion: 443–9].

3. Piolanti M, Coppola F, Papa S, et al. Ultrasonographic localization of occult pulmonary nodules during video-assisted thoracic surgery. Eur Radiol 2003;13:2358–64.

4. Wada H, Anayama T, Hirohashi K, et al. Thoracoscopic ultrasonography for localization of subcentimetre lung nodulesdagger. Eur J Cardiothorac Surg 2015;49(2):690–7.

5. Miyoshi K, Toyooka S, Gobara H, et al. Clinical outcomes of short hook wire and suture marking system in thoracoscopic resection for pulmonary nodules. Eur J Cardiothorac Surg 2009;36:378–82.

6. Dendo S, Kanazawa S, Ando A, et al. Preoperative localization of small pulmonary lesions with a short hook wire and suture system: experience with 168 procedures. Radiology 2002;225:511–8.

7. Ciriaco P, Negri G, Puglisi A, et al. Video-assisted thoracoscopic surgery for pulmonary nodules: rationale for preoperative computed tomography-guided hookwire localization. Eur J Cardiothorac Surg 2004; 25:429–33.

8. Mack MJ, Shennib H, Landreneau RJ, et al. Techniques for localization of pulmonary nodules for thoracoscopic resection. J Thorac Cardiovasc Surg 1993;106:550–3.

9. Suzuki K, Shimohira M, Hashizume T, et al. Usefulness of CT-guided hookwire marking before video-assisted thoracoscopic surgery for small pulmonary lesions. J Med Imaging Radiat Oncol 2014;58:657–62.

10. Galetta D, Bellomi M, Grana C, et al. Radio-guided localization and resection of small or ill-defined pulmonary lesions. Ann Thorac Surg 2015;100: 1175–80.

11. Gonfiotti A, Davini F, Vaggelli L, et al. Thoracoscopic localization techniques for patients with solitary pulmonary nodule: hookwire versus radio-guided surgery. Eur J Cardiothorac Surg 2007;32:843–7.

12. Hajjar WM, Alnassar S, Almousa O, et al. Thoracoscopic resection of suspected metastatic pulmonary nodules after microcoil localization technique, a prospective study. J Cardiovasc Surg (Torino) 2014. [Epub ahead of print].

13. Finley RJ, Mayo JR, Grant K, et al. Preoperative computed tomography-guided microcoil localization of small peripheral pulmonary nodules: a prospective randomized controlled trial. J Thorac Cardiovasc Surg 2015;149:26–31.

14. Kha LT, Hanneman K, Donahoe L, et al. Safety and efficacy of modified preoperative lung nodule microcoil localization without pleural marking: a pilot study. J Thorac Imaging 2016;31(1):15–22.

15. Su TH, Fan YF, Jin L, et al. CT-guided localization of small pulmonary nodules using adjacent microcoil implantation prior to video-assisted thoracoscopic surgical resection. Eur Radiol 2015;25: 2627–33.

16. McConnell PI, Feola GP, Meyers RL. Methylene blue-stained autologous blood for needle localization and thoracoscopic resection of deep pulmonary nodules. J Pediatr Surg 2002;37:1729–31.

17. Yoshida J, Nagai K, Nishimura M, et al. Computed tomography-fluoroscopy guided injection of cyanoacrylate to mark a pulmonary nodule for thoracoscopic resection. Jpn J Thorac Cardiovasc Surg 1999;47:210–3.

18. Magistrelli P, D'Ambra L, Berti S, et al. Use of India ink during preoperative computed tomography localization of small peripheral undiagnosed pulmonary nodules for thoracoscopic resection. World J Surg 2009;33:1421–4.

19. Moon SW, Wang YP, Jo KH, et al. Fluoroscopy-aided thoracoscopic resection of pulmonary nodule localized with contrast media. Ann Thorac Surg 1999; 68:1815–20.

20. Kawanaka K, Nomori H, Mori T, et al. Marking of small pulmonary nodules before thoracoscopic resection: injection of lipiodol under CT-fluoroscopic guidance. Acad Radiol 2009;16:39–45.

21. Watanabe K, Nomori H, Ohtsuka T, et al. Usefulness and complications of computed tomography-guided lipiodol marking for fluoroscopy-assisted thoracoscopic resection of small pulmonary nodules: experience with 174 nodules. J Thorac Cardiovasc Surg 2006;132:320–4.

22. Mogi A, Yajima T, Tomizawa K, et al. Video-assisted thoracoscopic surgery after preoperative CT-guided lipiodol marking of small or impalpable pulmonary nodules. Ann Thorac Cardiovasc Surg 2015;21:435–9.

23. Vandoni RE, Cuttat JF, Wicky S, et al. CT-guided methylene-blue labelling before thoracoscopic resection of pulmonary nodules. Eur J Cardiothorac Surg 1998;14:265–70.

24. Krimsky WS, Minnich DJ, Cattaneo SM, et al. Thoracoscopic detection of occult indeterminate pulmonary nodules using bronchoscopic pleural dye marking. J Community Hosp Intern Med Perspect 2014;4.

25. Bolton WD, Howe H 3rd, Stephenson JE. The utility of electromagnetic navigational bronchoscopy as a localization tool for robotic resection of small pulmonary nodules. Ann Thorac Surg 2014;98:471–5 [discussion: 475–6].

26. Asano F, Shindoh J, Shigemitsu K, et al. Ultrathin bronchoscopic barium marking with virtual bronchoscopic navigation for fluoroscopy-assisted thoracoscopic surgery. Chest 2004;126:1687–93.

27. Miyoshi T, Kondo K, Takizawa H, et al. Fluoroscopy-assisted thoracoscopic resection of pulmonary nodules after computed tomography–guided bronchoscopic metallic coil marking. J Thorac Cardiovasc Surg 2006;131:704–10.

28. Zaman M, Bilal H, Woo CY, et al. In patients undergoing video-assisted thoracoscopic surgery excision, what is the best way to locate a subcentimetre solitary pulmonary nodule in order to achieve successful excision? Interact Cardiovasc Thorac Surg 2012;15: 266–72.

29. Kidane B, Toyooka S, Yasufuku K. MDT lung cancer care: input from the surgical oncologist. Respirology 2015;20:1023–33.

30. Oizumi H, Endoh M, Takeda S, et al. Anatomical lung segmentectomy simulated by computed tomographic angiography. Ann Thorac Surg 2010;90: 1382–3.

31. Oizumi H, Kanauchi N, Kato H, et al. Anatomic thoracoscopic pulmonary segmentectomy under 3-dimensional multidetector computed tomography simulation: a report of 52 consecutive cases. J Thorac Cardiovasc Surg 2011;141:678–82.

32. Oizumi H, Kato H, Endoh M, et al. Techniques to define segmental anatomy during segmentectomy. Ann Cardiothorac Surg 2014;3:170–5.

33. Kanzaki M, Kikkawa T, Shimizu T, et al. Presurgical planning using a three-dimensional pulmonary model of the actual anatomy of patient with primary lung cancer. Thorac Cardiovasc Surg 2013; 61:144–50.

34. Ikeda N, Yoshimura A, Hagiwara M, et al. Three dimensional computed tomography lung modeling is useful in simulation and navigation of lung cancer surgery. Ann Thorac Cardiovasc Surg 2013;19:1–5.

35. Iwano S, Yokoi K, Taniguchi T, et al. Planning of segmentectomy using three-dimensional computed tomography angiography with a virtual safety margin: technique and initial experience. Lung Cancer 2013;81:410–5.

36. Nakada T, Akiba T, Inagaki T, et al. Thoracoscopic anatomical subsegmentectomy of the right S2b + S3 using a 3D printing model with rapid prototyping. Interact Cardiovasc Thorac Surg 2014;19:696–8.

37. Zhang Z, Liao Y, Ai B, et al. Methylene blue staining: a new technique for identifying intersegmental planes in anatomic segmentectomy. Ann Thorac Surg 2015;99:238–42.

38. Oh S, Suzuki K, Miyasaka Y, et al. New technique for lung segmentectomy using indocyanine green injection. Ann Thorac Surg 2013;95:2188–90.

39. Sekine Y, Ko E, Oishi H, et al. A simple and effective technique for identification of intersegmental planes by infrared thoracoscopy after transbronchial injection of indocyanine green. J Thorac Cardiovasc Surg 2012;143:1330–5.

40. Misaki N, Chang SS, Igai H, et al. New clinically applicable method for visualizing adjacent lung segments using an infrared thoracoscopy system. J Thorac Cardiovasc Surg 2010;140:752–6.

41. Pardolesi A, Veronesi G, Solli P, et al. Use of indocyanine green to facilitate intersegmental plane identification during robotic anatomic segmentectomy. J Thorac Cardiovasc Surg 2014;148:737–8.

42. Kasai Y, Tarumi S, Chang SS, et al. Clinical trial of new methods for identifying lung intersegmental borders using infrared thoracoscopy with indocyanine

green: comparative analysis of 2- and 1-wavelength methods. Eur J Cardiothorac Surg 2013;44:1103–7.

43. Sato M, Aoyama A, Yamada T, et al. Thoracoscopic wedge lung resection using virtual-assisted lung mapping. Asian Cardiovasc Thorac Ann 2015;23:46–54.

44. Sato M, Yamada T, Menju T, et al. Virtual-assisted lung mapping: outcome of 100 consecutive cases in a single institute. Eur J Cardiothorac Surg 2015;47:e131–9.

45. Sato M, Omasa M, Chen F, et al. Use of virtual assisted lung mapping (VAL-MAP), a bronchoscopic multispot dye-marking technique using virtual images, for precise navigation of thoracoscopic sublobar lung resection. J Thorac Cardiovasc Surg 2014;147:1813–9.

Novel Technologies for Isolated Lung Perfusion
Beyond Lung Transplant

Marcelo Cypel, MD*, Shaf Keshavjee, MD

KEYWORDS

- Lung perfusion • In vivo • Ex vivo • High-dose chemotherapy

KEY POINTS

- Strategies of isolated lung perfusion have been investigated for many years; however, significant progress has been made in recent years with lessons learned from lung transplantation and improvements in technology and lung perfusion solutions.
- EVLP has had a dramatic impact on clinical lung transplantation and a large body of research is being performed toward further technical optimizations and adjunct therapeutic strategies to repair donor organs.
- Advanced techniques of in vivo and ex vivo lung repair with gene and stem cell strategies using these perfusion technologies are now being investigated.

INTRODUCTION

Isolated lung perfusion (ILP) has been historically used as a method to study concepts of basic lung physiology using animal models. More recently, ILP has been further examined and developed in lung transplantation and thoracic oncology research. In lung transplantation, ILP has been used to assess physiologic integrity of donor lungs after removal from the donor. This procedure is called ex vivo lung perfusion (EVLP), and it has also been proposed as a method for active treatment and repair injured unsuitable donor organs ex vivo. Beyond lung transplantation, ILP has been primarily explored in thoracic oncology. ILP is attractive as a concept to potentially deliver high-dose chemotherapy to treat pulmonary metastatic disease. Because the lung vasculature is isolated in vivo, we refer to this technique as in vivo lung perfusion (IVLP). This article focuses on the rationale, technical aspects, and experimental and clinical experience of IVLP. A perspective on the future application of these techniques is described.

GENERAL CONCEPTS OF ISOLATED LUNG PERFUSION

Most of the knowledge in ILP has emerged from studies using organ perfusion ex vivo. EVLP simulates the in vivo scenario with ventilation and perfusion of the donor lung graft. In 1885, Max von Frey (1852–1932), while working at the Carl Ludwig Physiologic Institute in Leipzig, Germany, designed an apparatus that had criteria characteristic of a heart-lung machine. With this device, he perfused the entire lower extremity of dogs, and took measurements of oxygen consumption, and carbon dioxide and lactate production.[1] Originally proposed in 1938 by Carrel for organs in general[2] and then in 1970 by Jirsch and colleagues for the evaluation and preservation of lungs for distant

Financial Disclosure: M. Cypel and S. Keshavjee are cofounders of Perfusix Inc and XOR Labs Toronto.
Division of Thoracic Surgery, Department of Surgery, Toronto General Hospital, UHN, University of Toronto, 200 Elizabeth Street, 9N-969, Toronto, Ontario M5G 2C4, Canada
* Corresponding author.
E-mail address: marcelo.cypel@uhn.ca

procurement, attempts in those eras failed because of an inability to maintain the air-fluid barrier within the lung, leading to the development of edema and increased pulmonary vascular resistance in the donor lung during EVLP.[3] Driven by the objective to better evaluate lungs from donors after cardiocirculatory arrest, Steen and colleagues[4] in Lund, Sweden developed a modern ex vivo perfusion system with the intent of short-term evaluation of lung function of this population of lungs ex vivo. In doing so, they developed a buffered, extracellular solution with an optimal colloid osmotic pressure to act as the lung perfusate (Steen Solution, XVIVO Perfusion, Göteburg, Sweden). This solution helps hold fluid within the intravascular space during perfusion and provides some nutrients needed to maintain lung viability. The composition of Steen solution is a modification on the current clinically used preservation solution of low-potassium dextran glucose (Perfadex, XVIVO Perfusion) with human albumin as the major additional constituent. This protein is added primarily to maintain a higher oncotic pressure to reduce the development of pulmonary edema during perfusion. Steen and colleagues[4] used this solution mixed with red blood cells in combination with their circuit and were able to successfully perfuse and evaluate lungs in a large animal model for 1 hour without the development of pulmonary edema and subsequent successful transplantation. The ultimate goal of Steen's studies was to use EVLP as a method for short-term lung evaluation and thus the perfusion times were short. For the application of EVLP for extended preservation, improved evaluation, and the even loftier goals of lung recovery and repair, much more time is required.

We first described successful long-term (12 hour) EVLP using a lung-protective strategy for acellular normothermic perfusion and ventilation.[5] The strategies described next are relevant physiologic concepts for IVLP and EVLP. To achieve stable prolonged perfusion, several key lung protective strategies were used.[5] First, an acellular perfusate was used. Oxygen delivery to cells in the lung can occur via the airways (ventilator) and via the vasculature. This concept is also supported by previous studies where ventilation of a donor lung with room air at normothermia was demonstrated to preserve cell viability for many hours.[6,7] Acellular perfusion is logistically simpler for clinical use and also avoids the problem of limited lifespan of red blood cells in environment of the perfusion circuit.

Second, rather than subject the lungs to perfusion at 100% of cardiac output, maximal circuit flow was limited to 40%. This lower flow is protective in that it aids in the reduction of hydrostatic edema caused by perfusion and, despite lower flows to nondependent areas of the lung, histology and posttransplant function in EVLP lungs were shown to be normal. Third, we found that maintenance of a positive left atrial pressure of 3 to 5 mm Hg to be important for the success of long-term perfusion. This small, but positive left atrium (LA) pressure tents open the capillaries and postcapillary venules and prevents collapse of the microvessels from occurring during periods of increased in airway pressure and decreased flow that occur with alveolar distention during inspiration.[8] Absence of positive LA pressures can lead to unstable alveolar geometry and results in decreased lung compliance.[9]

Finally, we noted the importance of using a centrifugal pump. With ventilation, distention of the alveoli places pressure on the perialveolar vessels leading to cyclical increases in pulmonary vascular resistance with every breath. As a consequence of how a centrifugal pump functions, increased afterload to the pump results in decreased rotation and flow. Thus, the pump backs off during times of increased resistance rather than forcing fluid through, potentially causing injury or edema as a roller pump would do. During perfusion, oxygen is removed and carbon dioxide is added via a membrane oxygenator, essentially as a simulation of cellular metabolism. Removal of oxygen enables the measurement of lung function by taking the difference between postlung and prelung perfusate P_{O_2}. The addition of carbon dioxide helps maintain the homeostatic pH stability and acid-base balance of the perfusate. Carbon dioxide seems to be a contributor to endothelial protection during ILP. Using this strategy, reproducible, safe 12-hour normothermic ex vivo perfusion has been demonstrated in porcine and human lungs and this strategy of EVLP has been shown to interrupt ischemic injury related to prolonged static cold ischemia. This has been well validated in human lung transplantation.[5,10,11] The general components of a modern ILP circuit are shown in **Fig. 1**.

THE EVOLVING ROLE OF ISOLATED LUNG PERFUSION IN THORACIC ONCOLOGY

An attractive potential application of ILP is IVLP for the purpose of delivering high-dose chemotherapy or other anticancer agents to the lungs to treat cancer metastases without exposing the rest of the body to these agents and their associated side effects. The development of pulmonary metastases is a common occurrence in patients with advanced cancer. The most frequent

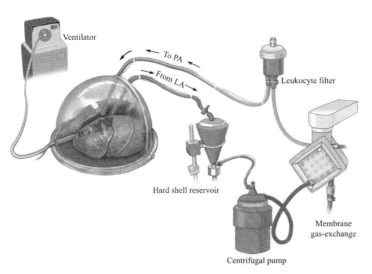

Fig. 1. Ex vivo lung perfusion system. LA, left atrium; PA, pulmonary artery. (*Adapted from* Cypel M, Keshavjee S. Ex vivo lung perfusion. J Thorac Dis 2014;6(8):1054–62; with permission.)

metastatic pulmonary diseases amenable to localized (lung) therapies originate from sarcomas and colorectal carcinoma because these malignancies often spread to lungs in isolation. Although surgical resection is a widely accepted treatment of pulmonary metastases, the 5-year survival rate of around 30% after complete resection remains disappointing.[12] Unfortunately, most patients develop recurrent disease even if complete resection is achieved, probably as a result of undetected micrometastatic disease present at the time of initial operation. Most recurrences occur in the lungs themselves, suggesting that the lung is the major reservoir of occult metastatic burden. The relatively poor results of surgical resection of pulmonary metastases combined with intravenous systemic chemotherapy are probably caused by drug resistance and the inability to achieve effective therapeutic drug concentrations within the lung.[13,14] This implies that better chemotherapeutic agents and more efficient drug delivery as an adjuvant to surgery are needed. IVLP provides the unique capability to selectively deliver an agent into the lung via the pulmonary artery and divert the venous effluent so that it is not systemically distributed. This allows a drug to be delivered in a higher dose locally in the lung, whereas drug levels in critical organs that are relatively sensitive to the drug are kept low enough to avoid severe side effects and toxicities (ie, hematologic, hepatic, cardiac, renal).

IVLP has been studied in animals and small clinical trials for more than 30 years. Although experimental studies have demonstrated remarkable efficacy, clinical translation has been impaired by technical challenges, high toxicity, and unconvincing oncologic benefits. With the development of

new perfusion technology, such as the current generation centrifugal pumps and membrane gas-exchangers, and a specific lung perfusion solution, a new wave in research in this area has emerged. Based on our expertise in EVLP, we have recently developed a new method of IVLP allowing safe in vivo normothermic perfusion for 4 hours without lung injury.[15] This technique is described next.

In Vivo Lung Perfusion Technique

In vivo lung perfusion circuit

The perfusate is circulated by a centrifugal pump passing through a leukocyte depletion filter and a membrane gas exchanger before entering the left lung through the pulmonary artery (**Fig. 2**). A filtered gas line for the gas exchange membrane is connected to a specialty gas mixture of oxygen (6%), carbon dioxide (8%), and nitrogen (86%). This mixture deoxygenates the perfusate and provides carbon dioxide to the inflow maintaining P_{CO_2} between 35 and 45 mm Hg (the gas flow is initiated at 1 L/min and adjusted to achieve the P_{CO_2} levels as mentioned). A heat exchanger is connected to the membrane gas exchanger to maintain the perfusate at 37°C. Pulmonary artery flow is controlled with the centrifugal pump and measured using an electromagnetic flow meter. The outflow perfusate returns from the pulmonary veins through the left atrial cannulas to a hard-shell reservoir. The height of the reservoir is used to control the left atrial pressure.

Priming the circuit

The reservoir of the circuit is primed with 1.5 L of Steen solution (XVIVO Perfusion). In addition to this, 500 mg of methylprednisolone, 1 g of

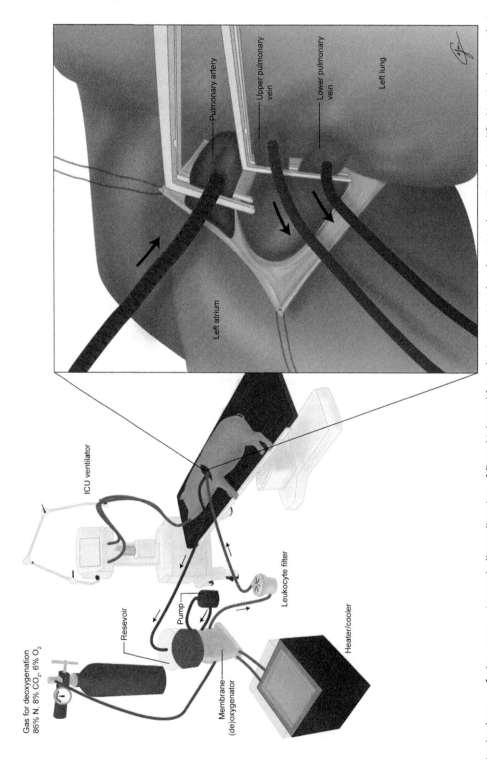

Fig. 2. In vivo lung perfusion system. *Arrows* indicate direction of flow. (*Adapted from* dos Santos PR, Iskender I, Machuca T, et al. Modified in vivo lung perfusion allows for prolonged perfusion without acute lung injury. J Thorac Cardiovasc Surg 2014;147:774–81; with permission.)

cefazolin, and 5000 IU of heparin are added to the perfusate.

Perfusion strategy

Perfusion is started at 37°C, with continuous measurement of the systemic, pulmonary artery, and LA pressures, with a flow established according to the estimated cardiac output. We use 20% of estimated cardiac output to perfuse each lung. To reach these rates, we use a strategy to gradually increase the flow, which consists of a three-step increment, starting with 30% of the calculated flow for 10 minutes, then moving to 60% for the next 10 minutes, and finally to 100% (at the full IVLP flow). Subsequently we adjust the reservoir height of the perfusion circuit to keep the LA pressure between 3 and 5 mm Hg.

Terminating in vivo lung perfusion and reperfusion phase

After IVLP, the venous cannulas are removed and a washout period is done in an anterograde fashion with 500 mL of a low-potassium dextran solution positioned 30 cm above the heart allowing passive drainage of the effluent through the left atrium by gravity. The purse string sutures in the pulmonary veins are then tied and the pulmonary artery clamp is removed.

Experimental Studies of In Vivo Lung Perfusion

Pulmonary metastases from sarcomas have been the most studied disease in the setting of IVLP. IVLP with doxorubicin in a methylcholanthrene-induced sarcoma model in the rat was found to be a safe and effective method, and superior to intravenous injection. With a perfusate drug concentration that was well tolerated by the animals, lung tissue doxorubicin levels were 20-fold higher than after intravenous injection.[16] After IVLP a complete clearance of macroscopic and microscopic tumor was observed, whereas sham perfused lungs had massive tumor replacement.[17] Perfusate doxorubicin concentration and the duration of perfusion were factors determining the final lung concentration of doxorubicin, whereas flow rate of perfusion did not influence tissue uptake.[18] In addition, this group compared six different perfusate solutions, and showed that low-potassium dextran solution[19] yielded the highest concentration of drug uptake in the lung tissue likely because of its capacity to recruit the pulmonary microcirculation.[18] Pulmonary artery pressures up to 25 mm Hg seem to be the maximum tolerated to prevent excessive lung damage with short-term IVLP.[20] Some studies also evaluated differences in tissue and tumor uptake with

retrograde and anterograde perfusion. Retrograde IVLP did not confer a better doxorubicin uptake in the tumor as compared with antegrade lung perfusion despite that the tumor vascularization in this model is greatly based on the bronchial artery circulation.[21] Johnston[22] provided a basis for further clinical and experimental studies by showing IVLP to be a safe technique in a large animal model.

Clinical Studies of In Vivo Lung Perfusion

In a pilot study by Johnston and colleagues[23] four patients with unresectable pulmonary metastatic sarcoma and four patients with diffuse bronchioloalveolar carcinoma were treated with doxorubicin and cisplatin via IVLP and cardiopulmonary bypass. Six patients were perfused with doxorubicin and two with cisplatin. Single left lung perfusion was performed in three patients and bilateral lung perfusion in five patients. Perfusion time ranged from 45 to 60 minutes at normothermic temperatures and whole blood was used as the perfusate. Pulmonary perfusate drug concentrations increased with higher doxorubicin dosages. Drug tissue levels also tended to increase with higher doses with only minimal systemic leakage. None of the eight patients had a partial or complete response to the regional chemotherapy and all died of progressive disease 23 to 151 days after lung perfusion. Burt and colleagues[24] described their results of IVLP with doxorubicin after extensive laboratory research. Eight patients with inoperable lung metastases from sarcoma underwent single lung perfusion in a phase I protocol. Intrapulmonary concentrations of doxorubicin correlated with the dose given, whereas systemic levels were minimal or undetectable. However, tumor levels were lower compared with lung levels. IVLP was performed in a deflated lung for 20 minutes using hetastarch plus blood as perfusate. The maximal tolerated dose (MTD) in this study was defined at 40 mg/m^2 of doxorubicin because a significant chemical pneumonitis developed in one patient at a dose of 80 mg/m^2. There were also no partial or complete responses. One patient had stabilization of disease in the perfused lung, whereas the lesions in the untreated lung progressed markedly. Putnam[25] reported another phase I study of isolated single-lung perfusion with doxorubicin in 16 patients with unresectable pulmonary metastatic disease, also patients with sarcoma. Systemic levels were minimal or undetectable, whereas two patients developed a grade 4 pulmonary toxicity at a dose of 75 mg/m^2, therefore defining the MTD at 60 mg/m^2 of doxorubicin in this study. Overall operative mortality was 18.8%. Only one major response occurred. Median survival time was 19.1 months in this study.

The group form Antwerp has recently translated their extensive laboratory work on IVLP to clinical trials. Their most recent phase I trial was performed using melphalan as the therapeutic agent in patients with resectable pulmonary metastases from sarcoma or colon cancer.[26] IVLP was performed for 30 minutes at the time of pulmonary metastatectomy. Hetastarch was used as the perfusate. In total, 21 procedures of ILP with complete metastatectomy were performed. Operative mortality was 0%, and no systemic toxicity was encountered. Grade 3 pulmonary toxicity developed at a dose of 60 mg of melphalan at 37°C and therefore 45 mg was defined as the MTD. An extension of this trial was performed using hyperthermic 42°C perfusion; however, pulmonary toxicity was significantly higher and therefore the authors recommended 37°C as the ideal temperature for IVLP.[27] A recent publication described long-term results of IVLP in the phase I melphalan trial. No major long-term pulmonary toxicity was observed and the 5-year overall and disease-free survival in this study was promising.[28]

Investigation of different perfusion techniques, including minimally invasive lung cannulation and perfusion techniques,[29] and the use of targeted molecular agents to treat cancer metastases to the lungs are major goals of the future. To that end, gene therapy to upregulate B7-1 (CD-80)[30] or interleukin-2[31] during IVLP are potential targets to treat and prevent osteosarcoma metastases to the lungs.

Other Techniques for Delivery of High-Dose Chemotherapy to the Lungs

Less invasive techniques have been proposed to achieve high concentrations of drugs in the lungs. The use pulmonary artery blood flow occlusion using a catheter-based technique has been recently proposed. Although the advantage of this technique is the avoidance of a thoracotomy, the potential disadvantage is the absence of lung isolation from systemic circulation and therefore systemic exposure to the drugs. In a study by Van Putte and colleagues,[32] significantly higher pulmonary gemcitabine peak concentrations were observed after gemcitabine and gemcitabine/carboplatin delivered by blood flow occlusion compared with intravenously, whereas no differences were shown between serum, renal, and lymph tissue.[33] Another described technique is chemoembolization using microspheres, which proved to be safe in a large animal model.[34]

Thoracoscopic pulmonary suffusion (temporary thoracoscopic pulmonary vein occlusions and fluoroscopy-guided transfemoral intravascular balloon occlusion of pulmonary artery) has also been described by Demmy and colleagues[35] in a small case series.

SUMMARY AND FUTURE PERSPECTIVES

Strategies of ILP have been investigated for many years; however, significant progress has been made in recent years with lessons learned from lung transplantation and improvements in technology and lung perfusion solutions. EVLP has had a dramatic impact in clinical lung transplantation and a large body of research is being performed toward further technical optimizations and adjunct therapeutic strategies to repair donor organs. Exciting spin-offs from the development of these novel perfusion technologies have opened the door to the revisitation of IVLP for the treatment of cancer metastases to the lung, and to the use of EVLP as a bioreactor for decellularization-recellularization and regeneration of lungs.[36,37] Finally, advanced techniques of in vivo lung repair with gene and stem cell strategies using these perfusion technologies are now being investigated.

REFERENCES

1. Zimmer HG. Perfusion of isolated organs and the first heart-lung machine. Can J Cardiol 2001;17:963–9.
2. Jirsch DW, Fisk RL, Couves CM. Ex vivo evaluation of stored lungs. Ann Thorac Surg 1970;10:163–8.
3. Carrel A, Lindbergh CA. The culture of whole organs. Science 1935;81:621–3.
4. Steen S, Liao Q, Wierup PN, et al. Transplantation of lungs from non-heart-beating donors after functional assessment ex vivo. Ann Thorac Surg 2003;76:244–52 [discussion: 52].
5. Cypel M, Yeung JC, Hirayama S, et al. Technique for prolonged normothermic ex vivo lung perfusion. J Heart Lung Transplant 2008;27:1319–25.
6. D'Armini AM, Roberts CS, Griffith PK, et al. When does the lung die? I. Histochemical evidence of pulmonary viability after "death". J Heart Lung Transplant 1994;13:741–7.
7. Alessandrini F, D'Armini AM, Roberts CS, et al. When does the lung die? II. Ultrastructural evidence of pulmonary viability after "death". J Heart Lung Transplant 1994;13:748–57.
8. Petak F, Habre W, Hantos Z, et al. Effects of pulmonary vascular pressures and flow on airway and parenchymal mechanics in isolated rat lungs. J Appl Physiol (1985) 2002;92:169–78.

9. Broccard AF, Vannay C, Feihl F, et al. Impact of low pulmonary vascular pressure on ventilator-induced lung injury. Crit Care Med 2002;30:2183–90.

10. Cypel M, Rubacha M, Yeung J, et al. Normothermic ex vivo perfusion prevents lung injury compared to extended cold preservation for transplantation. Am J Transplant 2009;9:2262–9.

11. Cypel M, Liu M, Rubacha M, et al. Functional repair of human donor lungs by IL-10 gene therapy. Sci Transl Med 2009;1:4ra9.

12. Pastorino U, McCormack PM, Ginsberg RJ. A new staging proposal for pulmonary metastases. The results of analysis of 5206 cases of resected pulmonary metastases. Chest Surg Clin N Am 1998;8:197–202.

13. Ranney DF. Drug targeting to the lungs. Biochem Pharmacol 1986;35:1063–9.

14. Hendriks JM, Van Putte BP, Grootenboers M, et al. Isolated lung perfusion for pulmonary metastases. Thorac Surg Clin 2006;16:185–98, vii.

15. dos Santos PR, Iskender I, Machuca T, et al. Modified in vivo lung perfusion allows for prolonged perfusion without acute lung injury. J Thorac Cardiovasc Surg 2014;147:774–81 [discussion: 81–2].

16. Weksler B, Ng B, Lenert JT, et al. Isolated single-lung perfusion with doxorubicin is pharmacokinetically superior to intravenous injection. Ann Thorac Surg 1993;56:209–14.

17. Weksler B, Lenert J, Ng B, et al. Isolated single lung perfusion with doxorubicin is effective in eradicating soft tissue sarcoma lung metastases in a rat model. J Thorac Cardiovasc Surg 1994;107:50–4.

18. Weksler B, Ng B, Lenert JT, et al. Isolated single-lung perfusion: a study of the optimal perfusate and other pharmacokinetic factors. Ann Thorac Surg 1995;60:624–9.

19. Keshavjee SH, Yamazaki F, Yokomise H, et al. The role of dextran 40 and potassium in extended hypothermic lung preservation for transplantation. J Thorac Cardiovasc Surg 1992;103:314–25.

20. Franke UF, Wittwer T, Lessel M, et al. Evaluation of isolated lung perfusion as neoadjuvant therapy of lung metastases using a novel in vivo pig model: I. Influence of perfusion pressure and hyperthermia on functional and morphological lung integrity. Eur J Cardiothorac Surg 2004;26:792–9.

21. Krueger T, Kuemmerle A, Andrejevic-Blant S, et al. Antegrade versus retrograde isolated lung perfusion: doxorubicin uptake and distribution in a sarcoma model. Ann Thorac Surg 2006;82:2024–30.

22. Johnston MR. Lung perfusion and other methods of targeting therapy to lung tumors. Chest Surg Clin N Am 1995;5:139–56.

23. Johnston MR, Minchen RF, Dawson CA. Lung perfusion with chemotherapy in patients with unresectable metastatic sarcoma to the lung or diffuse bronchioloalveolar carcinoma. J Thorac Cardiovasc Surg 1995;110:368–73.

24. Burt ME, Liu D, Abolhoda A, et al. Isolated lung perfusion for patients with unresectable metastases from sarcoma: a phase I trial. Ann Thorac Surg 2000;69:1542–9.

25. Putnam JB Jr. New and evolving treatment methods for pulmonary metastases. Semin Thorac Cardiovasc Surg 2002;14:49–56.

26. Hendriks JM, Grootenboers MJ, Schramel FM, et al. Isolated lung perfusion with melphalan for resectable lung metastases: a phase I clinical trial. Ann Thorac Surg 2004;78:1919–26 [discussion: 26–7].

27. Grootenboers MJ, Hendriks JM, van Boven WJ, et al. Pharmacokinetics of isolated lung perfusion with melphalan for resectable pulmonary metastases, a phase I and extension trial. J Surg Oncol 2007;96:583–9.

28. Den Hengst WA, van Putte BP, Hendriks JM, et al. Long-term survival of a phase I clinical trial of isolated lung perfusion with melphalan for resectable lung metastases. Eur J Cardiothorac Surg 2010;38:621–7.

29. Jinbo M, Ueda K, Kaneda Y, et al. Video-assisted transcatheter lung perfusion regional chemotherapy. Eur J Cardiothorac Surg 2005;27:1079–82.

30. Tsuji H, Kawaguchi S, Wada T, et al. Adenovirus-mediated in vivo B7-1 gene transfer induces anti-tumor immunity against pre-established primary tumor and pulmonary metastasis of rat osteosarcoma. Cancer Gene Ther 2002;9:747–55.

31. Sorenson BS, Banton KL, Frykman NL, et al. Attenuated salmonella typhimurium with interleukin 2 gene prevents the establishment of pulmonary metastases in a model of osteosarcoma. J Pediatr Surg 2008;43:1153–8.

32. van Putte BP, Grootenboers M, van Boven WJ, et al. Selective pulmonary artery perfusion for the treatment of primary lung cancer: improved drug exposure of the lung. Lung Cancer 2009;65:208–13.

33. Grootenboers MJ, Schramel FM, van Boven WJ, et al. Selective pulmonary artery perfusion followed by blood flow occlusion: new challenge for the treatment of pulmonary malignancies. Lung Cancer 2009;63:400–4.

34. Pohlen U, Rieger H, Albrecht T, et al. Chemoembolization with carboplatin of the lung. Feasibility and toxicity in a pig model. Anticancer Res 2007;27:1503–8.

35. Demmy TL, Tomaszewski G, Dy GK, et al. Thoracoscopic organ suffusion for regional lung chemotherapy (preliminary results). Ann Thorac Surg 2009;88:385–90 [discussion: 90–1].

36. Ott HC, Clippinger B, Conrad C, et al. Regeneration and orthotopic transplantation of a bioartificial lung. Nat Med 2010;16:927–33.

37. Petersen TH, Calle EA, Zhao L, et al. Tissue-engineered lungs for in vivo implantation. Science 2010;329:538–41.

Per Oral Endoscopic Myotomy for Achalasia
A Detailed Description of the Technique and Review of the Literature

Kevin L. Grimes, MD[a],*, Haruhiro Inoue, MD, PhD[b]

KEYWORDS

- Achalasia • Per oral endoscopic myotomy (POEM) • Technique

KEY POINTS

- POEM is performed safely and effectively in a wide range of patients, including pediatric patients and the elderly. In addition to classic achalasia, POEM is performed in cases of spastic esophageal motility disorders, advanced sigmoid achalasia, or following prior endoscopic or surgical treatment.
- Clinical results are excellent in short- and long-term follow-up and seem to be comparable or better than surgical myotomy.
- The technical points presented aid in the safe completion of the procedure and help reduce the risk of adverse events.
- Adjuncts to POEM, such as addition of a second endoscope, fluoroscopy, or EndoFLIP, help ensure a complete gastric myotomy and may reduce the risk of treatment failure.

INTRODUCTION

Achalasia is a spastic esophageal motility disorder characterized by loss of peristalsis and impaired relaxation of the lower esophageal sphincter (LES). The incidence may be up to 1 in 10,000, and patients typically present with progressive dysphagia and regurgitation of esophageal contents, weight loss, or chest pain. Historically, treatment has been aimed at reducing the resting pressure of the LES, including oral nitrates or calcium channel blockers, endoscopic pneumatic dilation or injection of botulinum toxin, or surgical myotomy. The most robust outcomes were seen with surgical myotomy.

Per oral endoscopic myotomy (POEM), first performed by our group in 2008, introduced an endoscopic method for creating a surgical myotomy.[1] Since that time, thousands of cases of POEM have been performed; however, there is no standard technique, and the rates of clinical success and adverse events vary widely among centers. Herein, we describe our technique in depth and analyze the benefits and potential pitfalls of published variations.

SURGICAL TECHNIQUE
Preoperative Planning

Diagnosis

Definitive diagnosis of achalasia is made by demonstrating an integrated relaxation pressure of 15 mm Hg or greater on high-resolution esophageal manometry, which has a sensitivity of 97%.[2] High-resolution esophageal manometry can differentiate three subtypes of achalasia, and identify other esophageal motility disorders that may respond to POEM (**Table 1**).[3]

Barium esophagram may demonstrate a classic "bird's beak" taper at the esophagogastric

[a] Department of Surgery, MetroHealth Medical Center, H924 2500 MetroHealth Drive, Cleveland, OH 44109-1998, USA; [b] Digestive Disease Center, Showa University Koto-Toyosu Hospital, Toyosu 5-1-38, Koto-ku, Tokyo 135-8577, Japan
* Corresponding author.
E-mail address: kevin.grimes@gmail.com

Thorac Surg Clin 26 (2016) 147–162
http://dx.doi.org/10.1016/j.thorsurg.2015.12.003
1547-4127/16/$ – see front matter © 2016 Elsevier Inc. All rights reserved.

Table 1
Selected esophageal motility disorders

Diagnosis	Peristalsis	Criteria
Achalasia	—	*IRP ≥15*
Type I (classic)	Absent	No additional criteria
Type II (panpressurization)	Abnormal	≥20% panpressurization
Type III (vigorous)	Abnormal	≥20% spastic contractions
EGJ outflow obstruction	Intact or weak	IRP ≥15
DES	Absent	Normal IRP, ≥20% premature contractions
Jackhammer esophagus	Absent	Normal IRP, DCI >8000
Nutcracker esophagus	Abnormal	Normal IRP, DCI >5000

Abbreviations: DCI, distal contractile integral (mm Hg-sec-cm); DES, diffuse esophageal spasm; EGJ, esophagogastric junction; IRP, integrated relaxation pressure (mm Hg).

junction (EGJ) and is useful in identifying dilation, sigmoid change, or diverticulum of the esophagus. Computed tomography (CT) of the chest may further subdivide sigmoid esophagus into type S1 (sigmoid change with one esophageal lumen on axial slices) and type S2 ("double" esophageal lumen on some slices), and exclude extrinsic compression from masses that may mimic achalasia.

Upper endoscopy may reveal stasis esophagitis or fungal overgrowth that should be treated preoperatively, and helps to exclude other causes of pseudoachalasia, such as submucosal nodules.

Contraindications
POEM has been safely performed in patients 3 years old and weighing 15 kg.[4] There is no upper age limit, provided the patient is healthy enough to tolerate a procedure.

There are few absolute contraindications. POEM should not be performed in patients with an inability to tolerate general anesthesia (eg, pulmonary disease), coagulopathy, portal hypertension, or prior radiation, ablation, or mucosal resection in the planned operative field, because of an increased risk of perforation or uncontrolled bleeding.[5]

Treatment of fungal infection
We treat only patients with overt evidence of fungal overgrowth. Some centers administer empiric fluconazole or nystatin in all patients for 2 to 3 days before the procedure, based on the high rate of esophageal stasis.[6,7]

Preparation and Patient Positioning

Endoscopy equipment
POEM is performed with a standard gastroscope; however, addition of an auxiliary water jet (eg, Olympus GIF-Q260J, Tokyo, Japan) and a distal attachment help to maintain a clear operative field, facilitate dissection, and protect against inadvertent thermal injury to surrounding structures. We prefer a straight hood (short ST, FujiFilm DH-28GR, Tokyo, Japan), but many centers use an oblique cap (Olympus MH-588, Tokyo, Japan).

Carbon dioxide insufflation should be used, because there is a higher risk of insufflation-related complications with room air.[8] There also seems to be a direct correlation between the flow rate and the rate of insufflation-related complications, with low-flow CO_2 tubing demonstrating the lowest rates of complications.[9] We also recommend careful control of insufflation by the endoscopist during the procedure.

Premedication
Intravenous antibiotics are administered preoperatively.[10] Most centers use a cephalosporin or a fluoroquinolone; we prefer cefazolin (or clindamycin in patients allergic to penicillin) based on the antimicrobial prophylaxis guidelines, treating POEM as a noncardiac thoracic procedure.[11] There is, however, no specific recommendation for or against the use of antibiotics during POEM.

We also administer an intravenous proton pump inhibitor (PPI) preoperatively, noting that more than half of patients may develop post-POEM reflux.[12]

Preparation of the esophagus
Many centers place patients on a liquid diet in the days before the POEM procedure to minimize residual esophageal contents.[5] Immediately before induction of anesthesia, esophagoscopy is performed to aspirate any residual contents and reduce the risk of aspiration.

Choice of anesthetic
We perform POEM under general endotracheal anesthesia. We believe that cuffed endotracheal

tubes help protect against aspiration, and that positive intrathoracic pressure may reduce the incidence of capnomediastinum and capnothorax.

A few cases have been reported using intravenous sedation, resulting in longer procedure times and increased complications, including bleeding, mucosal perforation, and pneumothorax.[8]

Patient position

The procedure is performed in either supine or left lateral decubitus positions. If a posterior myotomy is performed in the supine position, fluid may pool and obscure the operative field; however, left lateral positioning may exacerbate the anatomic distortions in patients with advanced sigmoid achalasia, increasing the difficulty of the procedure. We prefer the supine position, particularly for difficult cases. It is possible, although cumbersome, to change positions during the case if necessary.

Abdominal exposure

In a meta-analysis of 29 studies and 1045 patients, capnoperitoneum was noted in 16% of cases, with much higher rates in some individual studies.[13] Given this risk, we keep the abdomen exposed throughout the procedure to monitor for tense capnoperitoneum and to facilitate abdominal decompression as necessary.

Procedural Approach

Inspection

In the proximal esophagus, extrinsic compression from the trachea (12 o'clock), left main bronchus, and aortic arch (anterolateral) can often be identified. Compression from the spine posteriorly (6 o'clock) generally extends for the entire length of the esophagus and may help to maintain orientation (**Fig. 1**).

The location of the EGJ is noted by measuring the distance from the incisors. Many patients demonstrate a tight area just proximal to the EGJ, and there may be slight resistance to passage of the endoscope (**Fig. 2**). This tightness should be noted for comparison after myotomy completion. The EGJ can also be examined in retroflexed view from the stomach. The squamocolumnar junction is often visible distal to an area of tightness that moves with the endoscope.

The endoscope is withdrawn and the esophagus carefully examined for contractions that appear vigorous and/or nonperistaltic (**Fig. 3**). Normal physiologic tightness is often noted in the proximal esophagus at the upper esophageal sphincter.

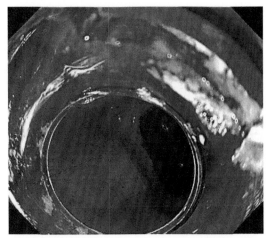

Fig. 1. Endoscopic view of the esophagus with external compression by the spine (*blue dashed lines*).

Selection of length

The point of entry depends on the planned length of the esophageal portion of the myotomy, which varies with the patient's diagnosis and findings of abnormal contractions during initial inspection. The mean length of the total myotomy (esophageal plus gastric) in published series ranges from 5.4 to 14.4 cm, with most centers clustering from 8 to 12 cm.[8,14]

As a default, the entry point is generally chosen 10 to 15 cm proximal to the EGJ, as first described by Inoue and colleagues.[1] This allows the tunnel to extend 2 to 3 cm proximal to the myotomy, which may protect against full-thickness perforation in the event of mucosal closure dehiscence.

A study by Teitelbaum and colleagues[15] examined the distensibility of the EGJ during POEM in 19 patients, suggesting a total myotomy length

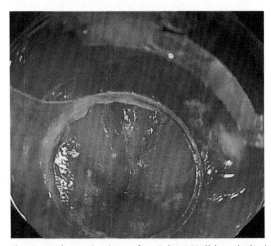

Fig. 2. Endoscopic view of a tight EGJ (*blue dashed circle*).

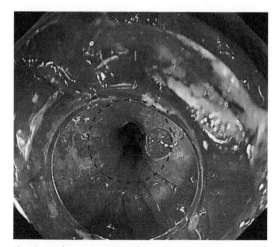

Fig. 3. Endoscopic view of an abnormal (nonperistaltic) esophageal contraction (*blue dashed circle*).

of 5 cm (3 cm gastric, 2 cm esophageal) may be sufficient for patients whose symptoms are attributable to tightness at the EGJ. This would be most applicable to Chicago type I (classic achalasia), type II (nonperistaltic panpressurization) without tight contractions proximally, or sigmoid achalasia with proximal dilation.

An extended proximal myotomy (up to 15 cm or more), however, is recommended for patients with Chicago type III (vigorous achalasia); type I or II with symptoms of chest pain and/or abnormal contractions on initial inspection; or spastic motility disorders, such as diffuse esophageal spasm or jackhammer esophagus.[16] This is consistent with literature that correlates noncardiac chest pain with sustained esophageal contractions and demonstrates the efficacy of extended surgical myotomy in relieving the pain.[17,18] Care should be taken to avoid disruption of the upper esophageal sphincter or injury to the trachea, left main bronchus, or aortic arch during extended proximal myotomy.

Selection of location
The procedure may be performed at any clock position. No studies have yet demonstrated a clear advantage of any specific location.

The initial description and first 500 cases by Inoue and colleagues[1,4] used a 2-o'clock (anterior) approach. Alternate anterior approaches include 11 o'clock and 12 o'clock.[5] The advantage of the anterior approach is avoidance of the gastric sling fibers, which may reduce the risk of post-POEM reflux; however, there may be an increased risk of bleeding from branches of the left gastric and left phrenic arteries.[19]

We currently favor the 5-o'clock (posterior) location. The advantages of this approach are

preservation of the anterior anatomy, which could allow for a straight-forward surgical myotomy in the future, and a theoretic decreased risk of bleeding because of fewer large blood vessels at this location. There is, however, a theoretic increased risk of post-POEM reflux if the gastric sling fibers are disrupted (**Fig. 4**).[19]

In selected cases, an 8-o'clock (greater curvature) myotomy may be indicated. Onimaru and colleagues[20] reported 21 cases of greater curvature myotomy, 17 of which had undergone Heller myotomy or prior POEM procedure. In this location, the angle of His serves as a consistent landmark for identification of the gastric side (**Fig. 5**), which is particularly useful in cases with distorted anatomy (sigmoid esophagus), fibrosis from a previous procedure (surgical Heller myotomy, lesser curvature myotomy, endoscopic submucosal dissection, and/or pneumatic balloon dilation), or inflammation from *Candida* esophagitis. The procedure is more technically challenging in the 8-o'clock position, and the main disadvantage is the high risk of post-POEM reflux caused by disruption of the angle of His. We believe greater curvature myotomy should be reserved for cases of redo-myotomy or cases with distorted anatomy that would make identification of the EGJ difficult.

Submucosal injection
After the starting point is chosen, a 25-gauge, 4-mm needle is used to perform "saline lift" by injecting fluid into the submucosal space (**Fig. 6**). This expands the potential space between the mucosa and the muscle fibers, which facilitates entry of the endoscope and protects against unintended myotomy. We prefer a solution of 500 mL of 5% dextrose in 0.45% NaCl with 20 mg of indigo

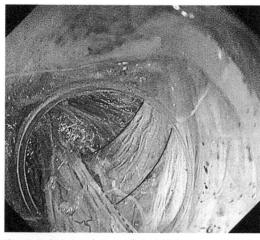

Fig. 4. Submucosal view of gastric sling muscle fibers (*blue dashed lines*) and circular muscle bundles (*solid black lines*).

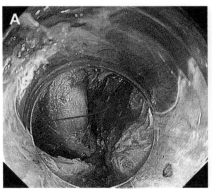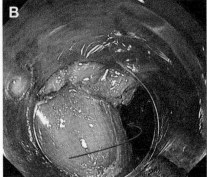

Fig. 5. (A, B) Submucosal views of the angle of His (blue arrows).

carmine dye, which helps to delineate the anatomy (submucosal fibers stain blue, whereas mucosa and muscle remain pink). This could also be performed with saline, a mixture of saline and alginate, or a mixture of 10% glycerol and 5% fructose. Methylene blue could be used in place of indigo carmine. We avoid solutions containing epinephrine because of the risk of cholinergic side effects.[19]

Mucosal incision

The mucosal incision is performed in a longitudinal direction to facilitate closure (Fig. 7). The mucosa is incised using a cutting current (eg, Endocut Q or Endocut I), and the submucosal fibers are dissected using spray coagulation until the circular muscle fibers are encountered. Full-thickness entry esophagotomy (Portland class I esophagotomy) has been reported, and care should be taken to avoid injury to the muscle layers.[21]

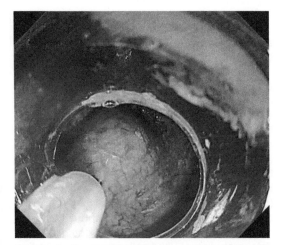

Fig. 6. Injection into the submucosal space with a 25-gauge 4-mm needle to perform a "saline lift" of the esophageal mucosa.

Creation of submucosal tunnel

Dissection of the submucosal space should be carried out close to the muscle fibers (Fig. 8). Any knife that can be used safely is acceptable. We divide submucosal fibers using the Triangle Tip (TT) knife (Olympus KD-640L, Tokyo, Japan) with spray coagulation (effect 2 at 50 W). Multiple submucosal injections are repeated as necessary using a blunt-tipped spray catheter (Olympus PW-5L-1, Tokyo, Japan) to ensure adequate working space and avoid injury to the backside of the mucosa (Fig. 9).

The Hybrid knife (ERBE 20150–060, Tübingen, Germany) may reduce the need for multiple instrument exchanges. In a study of 67 patients in China, the Hybrid knife reduced average procedure time by 15 minutes compared with the TT knife, and resulted in half as many instrument exchanges.[22]

The Hook knife (Olympus KD-620LR, Tokyo, Japan) can facilitate dissection when scarring or inflammation are encountered, or if the mucosal lift is insufficient for safe use of the TT knife (Fig. 10).

During dissection, perforating vessels may be encountered. Under normal circumstances, vessels on the esophageal side are controlled using the dissecting knife with a coagulating current. If neovascularization has occurred because of inflammation from Candida esophagitis or a prior procedure, the esophageal vessels may be larger and/or more frequently encountered. Larger vessels are controlled using a coagulating forceps (Coagrasper, Olympus FD-410LR, Tokyo, Japan) with a soft coagulation current (effect 5 at 80 W). On the gastric side, we prefer the coagulating forceps even for smaller vessels, because these tend to be difficult to control with the TT knife alone (Fig. 11).

Myotomy

The myotomy may be completed with a variety of knives, including the TT knife, the stag-beetle

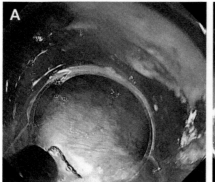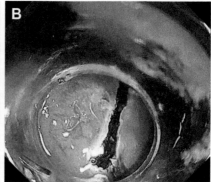

Fig. 7. Longitudinal mucosal incision with Triangle Tip (TT) knife using EndoCut electrical current. (*A*) during incision, and (*B*) after incision.

knife,[23] the Dual knife (Olympus KD-650L, Tokyo, Japan), the insulated tip knife (Olympus KD-611L, Tokyo, Japan), or the Hybrid knife. Anecdotal evidence suggests a selective circular myotomy may be technically easier to perform using the Hybrid knife to inject the intermuscular space, separating the circular and longitudinal fibers.

Anterograde esophageal myotomy begins 2 to 3 cm distal to the mucosal incision. This creates a short segment of intact mucosa overlying intact muscle, which protects against full-thickness perforation in the event of mucosal closure dehiscence. We prefer the TT knife, beginning with spray coagulation (effect 2 at 50 W) to control fine capillary vessels that run in the intermuscular space, then switching to cutting current (Endocut Q, effect 2, duration 1, interval 6) to divide the circular muscle bundles (**Fig. 12**). We find this technique provides adequate hemostasis

with minimal charring. The myotomy is carried for 2 to 3 cm onto the gastric cardia, where the muscle fibers assume an oblique orientation. Care should be taken to maintain a clear operative field with the needle tip in view at all times once the gastric cardia is reached. One case of massive bleeding has been reported because of inadvertent injury to a gastric perforating artery.[4]

Retrograde myotomy was reported by Ponsky and colleagues,[24] where the authors created a standard proximal to distal tunnel, then performed the myotomy in the distal to proximal direction. Outcomes were similar to the standard anterograde myotomy, but the most crucial part of the dissection (the EGJ) is performed earlier in case the procedure has to be aborted before completion of the myotomy. Our practice in cases where there is concern for the possibility of early termination of the procedure is to first divide the bundles at the EGJ (in an anterograde direction), then withdraw the endoscope to perform the proximal myotomy in standard fashion.

Studies have not demonstrated superiority of either selective (circular) or full-thickness (circular and longitudinal) myotomy. Full-thickness myotomy more closely recreates the surgical Heller myotomy, in which both muscle layers must be divided because of the extraluminal approach; however, in an international survey of POEM centers, only 12.5% of respondents preferred a full-thickness myotomy.[5] A small study by von Renteln and colleagues[25] found similar post-POEM Eckardt scores following selective and full-thickness myotomy. There are theoretic increases in the risks of insufflation-related adverse events (capnoperitoneum, capnomediastinum, or capnothorax) and post-POEM reflux with full-thickness myotomy, although the only direct comparison to date, a study by Li and colleagues,[26] did not find any statistically significant differences. Most of their cases, however, were performed with

Fig. 8. Endoscopic division of wispy submucosal fibers (*blue discoloration*) with pink circular muscle in the 6-o'clock position.

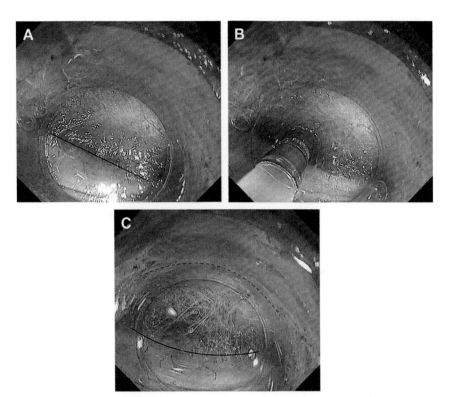

Fig. 9. Submucosal fluid injection. (*A*) Before injection, the circular muscle layer (*solid black line*) and backside of the mucosa (*dashed blue line*) are in close proximity. (*B*) Fluid injection with a blunt-tipped spray catheter. (*C*) After injection, the submucosal space is expanded, with adequate working distance between the circular muscle (*solid black line*) and the backside of the mucosa (*dashed blue line*).

air insufflation, which increases the rate of insufflation-related complications compared with CO_2.[27,28] We prefer a selective myotomy whenever technically possible.

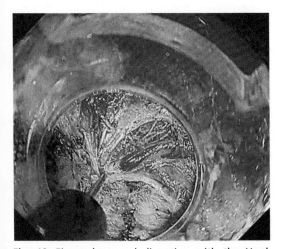

Fig. 10. Fine submucosal dissection with the Hook knife; fibrotic tissue is retracted away from a blood vessel.

Confirmation of adequate length

The main risk factor for clinical failure of POEM is an incomplete gastric myotomy. A gastric myotomy length of 2 to 3 cm is recommended based on a study by Oelschlager and colleagues,[29] which found improved outcomes during Heller myotomy when the gastric portion was extended from 1.5 cm to 3 cm.[10,30]

Endoscopic landmarks that are used to confirm adequate dissection onto the gastric cardia include distance markings on the endoscope, narrowing followed by widening of the submucosal tunnel, identification of pallisade vessels, and blue discoloration of the gastric mucosa on retroflexed view (**Fig. 13**); blue discoloration and narrowing followed by widening of the submucosal space are subjectively the most useful.[5] Endoscopic landmarks can be inaccurate, particularly in cases with distorted anatomy, scarring from prior procedures, or prior *Candida* esophagitis. Several adjuncts have been developed to ensure a complete gastric myotomy.

A technique described by Baldaque-Silva and colleagues[31] uses two endoscopes to verify the length of the submucosal tunnel by placing

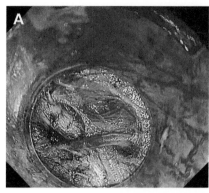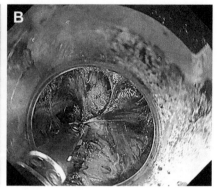

Fig. 11. A submucosal blood vessel (*A*) before and (*B*) during coagulation with a coagulating forceps using a "soft" coagulating current.

one endoscope in the tunnel and observing the transillumination with the second endoscope in retroflexed view of the gastric cardia (**Fig. 14**). A prospective study by Grimes and colleagues[32] randomized 100 patients to receive either single- or double-scope POEM and found that use of the second endoscope resulted in extension of the myotomy in 34% of cases and a significant increase in the average gastric myotomy length.

A second technique involves placement of a radiopaque clip to mark the EGJ, followed by fluoroscopy to measure the distance from the clip to the tip of the endoscope. A single-arm study of 24 patients by Kumbhari and colleagues[33] reported that the tunnel was extended in 21%.

A final technique uses EndoFLIP (Cropson Medical Devices, Galway, Ireland) to measure EGJ distensibility. Two studies have correlated low postprocedure distensibility with poor clinical outcomes.[34,35] Familiari and colleagues[36] used the system to guide decision-making during 23 POEM cases, extending the myotomy in one patient based on intraoperative readings.

We recommend the double-scope technique. Although there are no long-term data comparing standard POEM with any of the adjunct techniques, we find that endoscopic markers are inaccurate in a large proportion of cases. A second endoscope can be added with minimal increase in procedure time, no increase in morbidity, and no need for specialized training or equipment.

Mucosal closure

After confirming hemostasis, the mucosal incision may be closed with hemostatic clips (**Fig. 15**).[1] We find endoscopic clip closure is successful in most cases. When the mucosa is inflamed or macerated, addition of 20-mm endoloops (Olympus MAJ-340, Tokyo, Japan) helps to appose the mucosal edges (**Fig. 16**).[37]

Alternative methods of closure include endoscopic sutures (Overstitch, Apollo, Austin, TX), over-the-scope clips (Ovesco, Tübingen, Germany), or fully covered metal stents.[21,38–40] A small (n = 10) retrospective study comparing clips with sutures found faster closure time with clips, although the learning curve for suturing likely accounts for most of the difference; there was no significant difference in equipment costs.[41]

Immediate Postprocedural Care

Studies

Some centers obtain an immediate postoperative chest radiograph to exclude a significant capnothorax.[42] If CO_2 insufflation is used, small collections likely resorb spontaneously without clinical sequelae.

Before initiating oral intake, most centers obtain a water-soluble contrast esophagram on

Fig. 12. Selective circular myotomy performed with the TT knife; intact longitudinal muscle fibers (*dashed blue lines*) are seen after division of circular muscle bundles (*solid black line*).

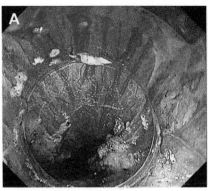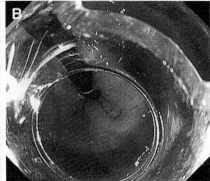

Fig. 13. Markers of the EGJ. (*A*) Submucosal view of palisade vessels (*dashed blue lines*) and (*B*) blue discoloration of the gastric mucosa (*dashed blue circle*) on retroflexed view of the cardia.

postoperative day (POD) 1 to exclude a leak and ensure smooth passage of contrast into the stomach. More than one-third of patients may demonstrate delayed esophageal emptying in the immediate postoperative period, but this does not portend long-term treatment failure.[43]

At our center, we also perform postoperative endoscopy to assess for partial-thickness mucosal necrosis (blanching) or development of a submucosal hematoma. If present, we delay oral intake for an additional 3 to 5 days until resolution is verified.

Postoperative CT scans are likely to demonstrate nonspecific inflammation or collections of gas that are considered normal postoperative findings; therefore, CT is not recommended in asymptomatic patients.[44]

Diet

Patients remain nothing-by-mouth status following the procedure. After studies to exclude mucosal

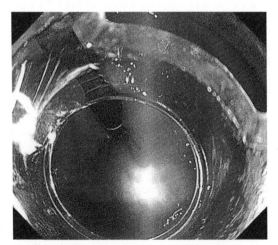

Fig. 14. Transillumination (*white spot*) from an endoscope in the submucosal tunnel, seen with a second endoscope on retroflexed view of the gastric cardia.

necrosis or esophageal leak, a liquid diet is initiated and continued for 1 week or more at some centers.[21] In patients who tolerate oral intake, we allow clear liquids on POD 1, pureed diet on POD 2 to 3, and regular diet on POD 4.

Medications

Normal postoperative pain control is instituted with parenteral opioids, which may be quickly de-escalated to over-the-counter nonsteroidal anti-inflammatory drugs or acetaminophen in many patients.

There is no consensus regarding the continuation of prophylactic antibiotics, which ranges from 24 hours up to 1 week postprocedure, depending on the center. The main concern is prevention of mediastinitis, although only four patients in the literature have required postoperative placement of drains, and there are no reported mortalities. We continue antibiotics until discharge on POD 4.

An oral PPI is continued for a minimum of 1 month, with some centers continuing indefinitely. We prescribe a PPI for 1 month, discontinue for 1 month, and then conduct the initial follow-up visit at 2 months postoperatively.[4]

Discharge

Patients may be discharged following a water-soluble contrast study, as early as POD 1.[7,42] Japanese patients stay in hospital until POD 4, mainly because of cultural differences and patient expectations.[4]

Follow-up

We conduct the initial follow-up visit at 2 months postoperatively, consisting of evaluation of the achalasia, including Eckardt score, esophageal manometry, and timed barium esophagram. We perform upper endoscopy to assess for esophagitis, and some centers may also include a pH

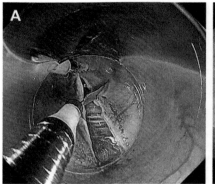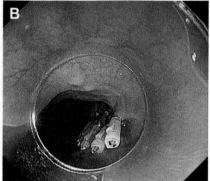

Fig. 15. Closure of the mucosal incision (*A*) during and (*B*) after approximation with hemostatic clips.

study.[4,7] We resume PPI based on the development of subjective symptoms of reflux or endoscopic findings of Los Angeles class C or D esophagitis.

We conduct subsequent follow-up, consisting of Eckardt score and esophagogastroduodenoscopy (EGD), at 1 year postoperatively and then annually.

CLINICAL RESULTS IN THE LITERATURE
Short-Term Outcomes (<2 Years)

Numerous studies, including two meta-analyses of more than 1000 patients each, have demonstrated the short-term success of POEM in reducing Eckardt scores and LES pressures.[13,45] Most centers report more than 90% clinical success rate, with a few rare exceptions, the lowest still being good at 82.4%.[46] Similar results are seen after prior surgical or endoscopic therapies; in pediatric patients; and in patients with spastic esophageal disorders, such as diffuse esophageal spasm or jackhammer esophagus.[6,16,20,47–51] Additionally, in a multicenter study involving 73 POEM patients, chest pain was significantly improved in 87%.[16]

Long-Term Outcomes (>2 Years)

Our center is the only group to date to report long-term clinical outcomes of the POEM procedure. Data from our first 500 cases demonstrated significant reductions in Eckardt scores and LES pressure, with an overall success rate of 88.5% at a minimum of 3 years' follow-up.[4]

Post Per Oral Endoscopic Myotomy Reflux

One of the main concerns with POEM, compared with laparoscopic Heller myotomy (LHM), is that an antireflux procedure is not performed

concurrently. The reported incidence of post-POEM reflux varies widely between series, from 5.7% in China to higher than 50% in America and Western Europe.[9,12,52,53] In two meta-analyses, the aggregate post-POEM reflux rates range from 10.9% to 19%, which is similar to the reflux rate of 8.8% to 17.4% observed following LHM.[13,45,54,55] In two studies comparing POEM with LHM, there was no statistically significant difference in the rates of reflux.[56,57]

A substantial number of patients, however, may be asymptomatic despite abnormal acid exposure. A study of 103 patients by Familiari and colleagues[58] found abnormal acid exposure in 50.5% of patients and esophagitis in 20.5% (including 5.8% with Los Angeles class C or D), although only 18.4% of patients reported symptoms. This is consistent with an earlier study by Jones and colleagues[59] that found no correlation between reflux symptom scores and acid exposure. We recommend long-term use of a PPI and/or continued endoscopic follow-up to monitor for the development of esophagitis in post-POEM patients. Our preference is ongoing endoscopic surveillance, and we use a PPI selectively in patients with subjective symptoms of reflux or Los Angeles class C or D esophagitis.

Comparison with Heller Myotomy

No randomized trials comparing POEM with LHM have yet been published. Four studies compared POEM with historical LHM controls, demonstrating similar complication rates and clinical success rates for both procedures. Operative times were similar or up to 30 minutes faster for POEM, and there was less blood loss, similar or lower postoperative pain, shorter length of hospital stay, and faster return to normal activity.[56,57,60,61]

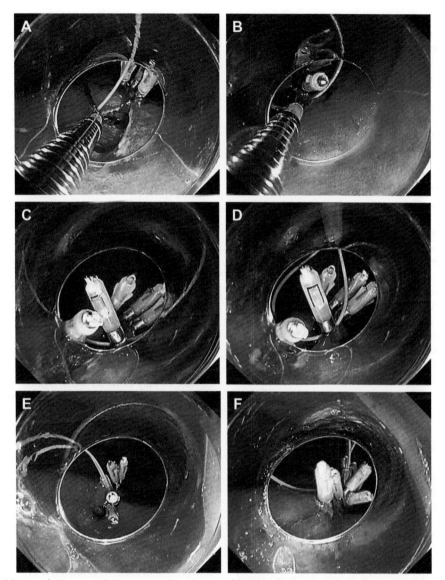

Fig. 16. Addition of 20-mm endoloops to aid in closure of thick, inflamed mucosa. (*A*) Clip fixation of the endoloop to the left mucosal edge. (*B*) Clip fixation of the endoloop to the right mucosal edge. (*C–E*) Tightening of the endoloop to approximate the mucosal edges. (*F*) Final mucosal closure after application of two endoloops.

Two studies by Teitelbaum and colleagues[15,62] demonstrated similar increases in EGJ distensibility following both POEM and LHM, although this is of uncertain clinical significance.

POTENTIAL COMPLICATIONS AND MANAGEMENT

Overall complication rates vary widely among centers and studies because of heterogeneity in definitions and reporting. Pooled analyses demonstrate adverse event rates that are similar to LHM.[13,45]

Insufflation-Related

Prevention
The most common adverse events are related to insufflation. In pooled analyses, the rates of capnoperitoneum (16.2%–30.6%), capnothorax (8.7%–11%), mediastinal emphysema (4.9%), and subcutaneous emphysema (21.8%–36.1%) were relatively high. However, only 8% of patients with capnoperitoneum and 2.7% of patients with capnothorax required decompression.[13,45] The rate seems to be technique-dependent; higher rates of insufflation-related events are seen with

air insufflation or high-flow CO_2.[8,9] We recommend CO_2 insufflation with low-flow tubing, combined with a conscious effort by the endoscopist to limit the insufflation to the minimum necessary for safe completion of the procedure.

There is a theoretic increase in the risk of insufflation-related events when a full-thickness myotomy is performed; however, in the only study comparing full-thickness with selective myotomy, no difference was found.[26]

Management

If air insufflation is used, pneumothorax may require tube thoracostomy for decompression. With CO_2 insufflation, however, capnothorax, capnomediastinum, and capnoperitoneum are generally self-limited and require no specific intervention. Tense capnoperitoneum can manifest with increased end-tidal CO_2 or increased ventilator peak pressures and poses a theoretic risk for abdominal compartment syndrome. The abdomen can be decompressed with an angiocatheter or Veress needle that is removed at the conclusion of the case. When abdominal decompression is necessary, we prefer to place an 18-gauge angiocatheter in the epigastric region after endoscopic decompression of the stomach.

Bleeding

Procedural

Minor bleeding commonly occurs and is controlled using a hemostatic forceps or the knife with a coagulating current. The Hybrid knife seems to reduce the number of minor bleeding episodes compared with standard dissection.[63]

One case of severe (arterial) bleeding was reported by Inoue and colleagues[4] early in their experience, but hemostasis was achieved using hemostatic forceps. There are no reported cases of procedural bleeding that could not be controlled endoscopically.

Delayed

Postprocedure bleeding occurs in 1% of cases.[13,45] Bleeding is generally self-limited; hemodynamically stable patients have been successfully managed with conservative treatment or following a diagnostic EGD without therapeutic intervention.[14,21,46,64] In one report, a patient on continuous antiplatelet therapy developed a submucosal hematoma postoperatively. The hematoma was followed with serial CT scans. The patient did well with conservative treatment, and was discharged on POD 8.[65]

There are reports of endoscopic procedures for bleeding, but none of the patients required operative intervention. In three cases, bleeding from the cut edge of the muscle was identified within the tunnel during EGD and controlled with hemostatic forceps.[66,67] In another case, clot was evacuated from the submucosal tunnel, but a source of bleeding could not be identified; a Sengstaken-Blakemore tube was inserted and left in place for 4 days, and the patient was discharged home 2 days later.[28] Of note, post-POEM patients are likely to have much higher risk of full-thickness perforation with inflation of an esophageal balloon because of the underlying muscle defect.

As a last resort, superselective coil embolization by interventional radiology may be an option.[68]

Perforation

The incidence of minor mucosal perforations is 2.6% in a pooled analysis, with some centers reporting accidental mucosotomy rates of 26%.[13,69] Most perforations are managed endoscopically during the procedure using clips with or without endoloops, fibrin glue, the Overstitch device, or fully covered metal stents.[70–73]

There are no reports of perforations that required open surgery. Minimally invasive drainage has been reported in four patients. One patient was noncompliant with her diet, retched, and developed a contained esophageal perforation at the EGJ. The defect could not be identified and laparoscopic drains were placed. She recovered well but ultimately developed a stricture and recurrent dysphagia.[60] Two patients had delayed full-thickness perforations that were not identified on routine postoperative imaging; one underwent thoracoscopic drainage, and the other was managed with endoscopic clips combined with percutaneous drainage of a pleural effusion.[61,67] The final patient developed a retroperitoneal abscess that was successfully treated with ultrasound-guided drainage and intravenous antibiotics.[67]

Postprocedure CT scans may demonstrate abnormal findings in a large percentage of patients, including pneumoperitoneum and/or pneumomediastinum (53.7%), subcutaneous emphysema (29.6%), pleural effusion (69.4%), atelectasis (29.6%), or minor pulmonary inflammation (69.4%).[67] There is no apparent correlation between pneumoperitoneum/pneumomediastinum and the development of complications, and these are considered normal postoperative findings in otherwise stable patients. Moderate pleural effusion or moderate ascites, however, may be predictive of severe complications, and may warrant further investigation.[67]

To reduce the risk of procedural and delayed perforation, the submucosal tunnel should be developed as close to the muscle as possible, maintaining adequate distance from the mucosa to avoid unintended thermal injury.

Aspiration

Esophageal stasis increases the risk of aspiration pneumonitis during general anesthesia. Only two cases of aspiration have been reported; both patients recovered following bronchial lavage and prolonged hospital stay.[32,74] Subclinical aspiration rates may be higher, because a large number of patients demonstrate pulmonary changes on post-POEM CT scans.[67] We recommend endoscopic aspiration of residual esophageal contents under light sedation immediately before the procedure, followed by performance of the procedure itself under general anesthesia with a cuffed endotracheal tube.

Leukopenia

Leukopenia is a rare side effect of PPIs that should be considered in post-POEM patients, who are almost universally administered a PPI perioperatively. One case of post-POEM leukopenia has been reported in an otherwise healthy 42-year-old woman, which resolved with discontinuation of her PPI.[32]

Death

No mortalities directly related to POEM have been reported. One death in a post-POEM patient was attributed to cachexia and considered a long-term treatment failure.[45]

SUMMARY

POEM is a safe and effective technique for the treatment of achalasia and spastic esophageal motility disorders, with excellent results in short- and long-term follow-up. The procedure has been successfully performed in children as young as 3 years, and in the elderly. Further studies are needed to establish the optimal length and location of the myotomy to ensure relief of dysphagia while minimizing the risk of post-POEM reflux. Ongoing randomized trials comparing POEM with LHM may ultimately establish POEM as the preferred treatment of achalasia.

REFERENCES

1. Inoue H, Minami H, Kobayashi Y, et al. Peroral endoscopic myotomy (POEM) for esophageal achalasia. Endoscopy 2010;42(4):265–71.

2. Kahrilas PJ, Peters JH. Evaluation of the esophagogastric junction using high resolution manometry and esophageal pressure topography. Neurogastroenterology Motil 2012;24(Suppl 1):11–9.

3. Bredenoord AJ, Fox M, Kahrilas PJ, et al. Chicago classification criteria of esophageal motility disorders defined in high resolution esophageal pressure topography. Neurogastroenterology Motil 2012; 24(Suppl 1):57–65.

4. Inoue H, Sato H, Ikeda H, et al. Per-oral endoscopic myotomy: a series of 500 patients. J Am Coll Surgeons 2015;221(2):256–64.

5. Stavropoulos SN, Modayil RJ, Friedel D, et al. The International Per Oral Endoscopic Myotomy Survey (IPOEMS): a snapshot of the global POEM experience. Surg Endosc 2013;27(9):3322–38.

6. Orenstein SB, Raigani S, Wu YV, et al. Peroral endoscopic myotomy (POEM) leads to similar results in patients with and without prior endoscopic or surgical therapy. Surg Endosc 2015;29(5):1064–70.

7. Sharata A, Kurian AA, Dunst CM, et al. Technique of per-oral endoscopic myotomy (POEM) of the esophagus (with video). Surg Endosc 2014;28(4):1333.

8. Wang J, Tan N, Xiao Y, et al. Safety and efficacy of the modified peroral endoscopic myotomy with shorter myotomy for achalasia patients: a prospective study. Dis esophagus 2014;28(8):720–7.

9. Familiari P, Gigante G, Marchese M, et al. Peroral endoscopic myotomy for esophageal achalasia: outcomes of the first 100 patients with short-term follow-up. Ann Surg 2016;263(1):82–7.

10. Stavropoulos SN, Desilets DJ, Fuchs KH, et al. Per-oral endoscopic myotomy white paper summary. Surg Endosc 2014;28(7):2005–19.

11. Bratzler DW, Dellinger EP, Olsen KM, et al. Clinical practice guidelines for antimicrobial prophylaxis in surgery. Surg Infect (Larchmt) 2013;14(1):73–156.

12. Verlaan T, Rohof WO, Bredenoord AJ, et al. Effect of peroral endoscopic myotomy on esophagogastric junction physiology in patients with achalasia. Gastrointest Endosc 2013;78(1):39–44.

13. Talukdar R, Inoue H, Reddy DN. Efficacy of peroral endoscopic myotomy (POEM) in the treatment of achalasia: a systematic review and meta-analysis. Surg Endosc 2015;29(11):3030–46.

14. Minami H, Isomoto H, Yamaguchi N, et al. Peroral endoscopic myotomy for esophageal achalasia: clinical impact of 28 cases. Dig Endosc 2014; 26(1):43–51.

15. Teitelbaum EN, Soper NJ, Pandolfino JE, et al. An extended proximal esophageal myotomy is necessary to normalize EGJ distensibility during Heller myotomy for achalasia, but not POEM. Surg Endosc 2014;28(10):2840–7.

16. Khashab MA, Messallam AA, Onimaru M, et al. International multicenter experience with peroral endoscopic myotomy for the treatment of spastic

esophageal disorders refractory to medical therapy (with video). Gastrointest Endosc 2015;81(5):1170–7.

17. Balaban DH, Yamamoto Y, Liu J, et al. Sustained esophageal contraction: a marker of esophageal chest pain identified by intraluminal ultrasonography. Gastroenterology 1999;116(1):29–37.

18. Leconte M, Douard R, Gaudric M, et al. Functional results after extended myotomy for diffuse oesophageal spasm. Br J Surg 2007;94(9):1113–8.

19. Bechara R, Ikeda H, Inoue H. Peroral endoscopic myotomy: an evolving treatment for achalasia. Nat Rev Gastroenterol Hepatol 2015;12(7):410–26.

20. Onimaru M, Inoue H, Ikeda H, et al. Greater curvature myotomy is a safe and effective modified technique in per-oral endoscopic myotomy (with videos). Gastrointest Endosc 2015;81(6):1370–7.

21. Sharata AM, Dunst CM, Pescarus R, et al. Peroral endoscopic myotomy (POEM) for esophageal primary motility disorders: analysis of 100 consecutive patients. J Gastrointest Surg 2015;19(1):161–70 [discussion: 170].

22. Tang X, Gong W, Deng Z, et al. Comparison of conventional versus Hybrid knife peroral endoscopic myotomy methods for esophageal achalasia: a case-control study. Scand J Gastroenterol 2016; 51(4):494–500.

23. Bittinger M, Messmann H. Use of the stag-beetle knife for peroral endoscopic myotomy for achalasia: a novel method for myotomy. Gastrointest Endosc 2015;82(2):401–2.

24. Ponsky JL, Marks JM, Orenstein SB. Retrograde myotomy: a variation in per oral endoscopic myotomy (POEM) technique. Surg Endosc 2014;28(11): 3257–9.

25. von Renteln D, Inoue H, Minami H, et al. Peroral endoscopic myotomy for the treatment of achalasia: a prospective single center study. Am J Gastroenterol 2012;107(3):411–7.

26. Li QL, Chen WF, Zhou PH, et al. Peroral endoscopic myotomy for the treatment of achalasia: a clinical comparative study of endoscopic full-thickness and circular muscle myotomy. J Am Coll Surgeons 2013;217(3):442–51.

27. Maeda Y, Hirasawa D, Fujita N, et al. A pilot study to assess mediastinal emphysema after esophageal endoscopic submucosal dissection with carbon dioxide insufflation. Endoscopy 2012;44(6):565–71.

28. Ren Z, Zhong Y, Zhou P, et al. Perioperative management and treatment for complications during and after peroral endoscopic myotomy (POEM) for esophageal achalasia (EA) (data from 119 cases). Surg Endosc 2012;26(11):3267–72.

29. Oelschlager BK, Chang L, Pellegrini CA. Improved outcome after extended gastric myotomy for achalasia. Arch Surg 2003;138(5):490–5 [discussion: 495–7].

30. Donahue PE, Teresi M, Patel S, et al. Laparoscopic myotomy in achalasia: intraoperative evidence for myotomy of the gastric cardia. Dis esophagus 1999;12(1):30–6.

31. Baldaque-Silva F, Marques M, Vilas-Boas F, et al. New transillumination auxiliary technique for peroral endoscopic myotomy. Gastrointest Endosc 2014; 79(4):544–5.

32. Grimes KL, Inoue H, Onimaru M, et al. Double-scope per oral endoscopic myotomy (POEM): a prospective randomized controlled trial. Surg Endosc 2015. [Epub ahead of print].

33. Kumbhari V, Besharati S, Abdelgelil A, et al. Intraprocedural fluoroscopy to determine the extent of the cardiomyotomy during per-oral endoscopic myotomy (with video). Gastrointest Endosc 2015; 81(6):1451–6.

34. Rohof WO, Hirsch DP, Kessing BF, et al. Efficacy of treatment for patients with achalasia depends on the distensibility of the esophagogastric junction. Gastroenterology 2012;143(2):328–35.

35. Pandolfino JE, de Ruigh A, Nicodeme F, et al. Distensibility of the esophagogastric junction assessed with the functional lumen imaging probe (FLIP) in achalasia patients. Neurogastroenterology Motil 2013;25(6):496–501.

36. Familiari P, Gigante G, Marchese M, et al. EndoFLIP system for the intraoperative evaluation of peroral endoscopic myotomy. United Eur Gastroenterol J 2014;2(2):77–83.

37. Zhang Y, Wang X, Fan Z. Reclosure of ruptured incision after peroral endoscopic myotomy using endoloops and metallic clips. Dig Endosc 2014; 26(2):295.

38. Saxena P, Chavez YH, Kord Valeshabad A, et al. An alternative method for mucosal flap closure during peroral endoscopic myotomy using an over-the-scope clipping device. Endoscopy 2013;45(7): 579–81.

39. Yang D, Draganov PV. Closing the gap in POEM. Endoscopy 2013;45(8):677.

40. Yang D, Zhang Q, Draganov PV. Successful placement of a fully covered esophageal stent to bridge a difficult-to-close mucosal incision during peroral endoscopic myotomy. Endoscopy 2014;46(Suppl 1 UCTN):E467–8.

41. Pescarus R, Shlomovitz E, Sharata AM, et al. Endoscopic suturing versus endoscopic clip closure of the mucosotomy during a per-oral endoscopic myotomy (POEM): a case-control study. Surg Endosc 2015. [Epub ahead of print].

42. Ponsky JL, Marks JM, Pauli EM. How I do it: per-oral endoscopic myotomy (POEM). J Gastrointest Surg 2012;16(6):1251–5.

43. Sternbach JM, El Khoury R, Teitelbaum EN, et al. Early esophagram in per-oral endoscopic myotomy (POEM) for achalasia does not predict long-term outcomes. Surgery 2015; 158(4):1128–35.

44. Cai MY, Zhou PH, Yao LQ, et al. Thoracic CT after peroral endoscopic myotomy for the treatment of achalasia. Gastrointest Endosc 2014;80(6): 1046–55.

45. Patel K, Abbassi-Ghadi N, Markar S, et al. Peroral endoscopic myotomy for the treatment of esophageal achalasia: systematic review and pooled analysis. Dis esophagus 2015. [Epub ahead of print].

46. Von Renteln D, Fuchs KH, Fockens P, et al. Peroral endoscopic myotomy for the treatment of achalasia: an international prospective multicenter study. Gastroenterology 2013;145(2):309–11.e1–3.

47. Vigneswaran Y, Yetasook AK, Zhao JC, et al. Peroral endoscopic myotomy (POEM): feasible as reoperation following Heller myotomy. J Gastrointest Surg 2014;18(6):1071–6.

48. Zhou PH, Li QL, Yao LQ, et al. Peroral endoscopic remyotomy for failed Heller myotomy: a prospective single-center study. Endoscopy 2013;45(3):161–6.

49. Sharata A, Kurian AA, Dunst CM, et al. Peroral endoscopic myotomy (POEM) is safe and effective in the setting of prior endoscopic intervention. J Gastrointest Surg 2013;17(7):1188–92.

50. Chen WF, Li QL, Zhou PH, et al. Long-term outcomes of peroral endoscopic myotomy for achalasia in pediatric patients: a prospective, single-center study. Gastrointest Endosc 2015;81(1):91–100.

51. Li C, Tan Y, Wang X, et al. Peroral endoscopic myotomy for treatment of achalasia in children and adolescents. J Pediatr Surg 2015;50(1):201–5.

52. Ling TS, Guo HM, Yang T, et al. Effectiveness of peroral endoscopic myotomy in the treatment of achalasia: a pilot trial in Chinese Han population with a minimum of one-year follow-up. J Dig Dis 2014;15(7):352–8.

53. Teitelbaum EN, Soper NJ, Santos BF, et al. Symptomatic and physiologic outcomes one year after peroral esophageal myotomy (POEM) for treatment of achalasia. Surg Endosc 2014;28(12):3359–65.

54. Wang L, Li YM, Li L. Meta-analysis of randomized and controlled treatment trials for achalasia. Dig Dis Sci 2009;54(11):2303–11.

55. Yaghoobi M, Mayrand S, Martel M, et al. Laparoscopic Heller's myotomy versus pneumatic dilation in the treatment of idiopathic achalasia: a meta-analysis of randomized, controlled trials. Gastrointest Endosc 2013;78(3):468–75.

56. Bhayani NH, Kurian AA, Dunst CM, et al. A comparative study on comprehensive, objective outcomes of laparoscopic Heller myotomy with per-oral endoscopic myotomy (POEM) for achalasia. Ann Surg 2014;259(6):1098–103.

57. Chan SM, Wu JC, Teoh AY, et al. Comparison of early outcomes and quality of life after laparoscopic Heller's cardiomyotomy to peroral endoscopic myotomy for treatment of achalasia. Dig Endosc 2016; 28(1):27–32.

58. Familiari P, Greco S, Gigante G, et al. Gastro-esophageal reflux disease after Per-Oral Endoscopic Myotomy (POEM). Analysis of clinical, procedural and functional factors, associated with GERD and esophagitis. Dig Endosc 2016;28(1):33–41.

59. Jones EL, Meara MP, Schwartz JS, et al. Gastro-esophageal reflux symptoms do not correlate with objective pH testing after peroral endoscopic myotomy. Surg Endosc 2015. [Epub ahead of print].

60. Hungness ES, Teitelbaum EN, Santos BF, et al. Comparison of perioperative outcomes between peroral esophageal myotomy (POEM) and laparoscopic Heller myotomy. J Gastrointest Surg 2013;17(2): 228–35.

61. Ujiki MB, Yetasook AK, Zapf M, et al. Peroral endoscopic myotomy: a short-term comparison with the standard laparoscopic approach. Surgery 2013; 154(4):893–7 [discussion: 897–900].

62. Teitelbaum EN, Boris L, Arafat FO, et al. Comparison of esophagogastric junction distensibility changes during POEM and Heller myotomy using intraoperative FLIP. Surg Endosc 2013;27(12):4547–55.

63. Cai MY, Zhou PH, Yao LQ, et al. Peroral endoscopic myotomy for idiopathic achalasia: randomized comparison of water-jet assisted versus conventional dissection technique. Surg Endosc 2014;28(4): 1158–65.

64. Kurian AA, Dunst CM, Sharata A, et al. Peroral endoscopic esophageal myotomy: defining the learning curve. Gastrointest Endosc 2013;77(5):719–25.

65. Benech N, Pioche M, O'Brien M, et al. Esophageal hematoma after peroral endoscopic myotomy for achalasia in a patient on antiplatelet therapy. Endoscopy 2015;47(Suppl 1):E363–4.

66. Li QL, Zhou PH, Yao LQ, et al. Early diagnosis and management of delayed bleeding in the submucosal tunnel after peroral endoscopic myotomy for achalasia (with video). Gastrointest Endosc 2013; 78(2):370–4.

67. Yang S, Zeng MS, Zhang ZY, et al. Pneumomediastinum and pneumoperitoneum on computed tomography after peroral endoscopic myotomy (POEM): postoperative changes or complications? Acta radiologica 2015;56(10):1216–21.

68. Vogten JM, Overtoom TT, Lely RJ, et al. Superselective coil embolization of arterial esophageal hemorrhage. J Vasc Interv Radiol 2007;18(6):771–3.

69. Patel KS, Calixte R, Modayil RJ, et al. The light at the end of the tunnel: a single-operator learning curve analysis for per oral endoscopic myotomy. Gastrointest Endosc 2015;81(5):1181–7.

70. Kurian AA, Bhayani NH, Reavis K, et al. Endoscopic suture repair of full-thickness esophagotomy during per-oral esophageal myotomy for achalasia. Surg Endosc 2013;27(10):3910.

71. Modayil R, Friedel D, Stavropoulos SN. Endoscopic suture repair of a large mucosal perforation

during peroral endoscopic myotomy for treatment of achalasia. Gastrointest Endosc 2014;80(6): 1169–70.

72. Ling T, Pei Q, Pan J, et al. Successful use of a covered, retrievable stent to seal a ruptured mucosal flap safety valve during peroral endoscopic myotomy in a child with achalasia. Endoscopy 2013; 45(Suppl 2 UCTN):E63–4.

73. Li H, Linghu E, Wang X. Fibrin sealant for closure of mucosal penetration at the cardia during peroral endoscopic myotomy (POEM). Endoscopy 2012; 44(Suppl 2 UCTN):E215–6.

74. Chiu PW, Wu JC, Teoh AY, et al. Peroral endoscopic myotomy for treatment of achalasia: from bench to bedside (with video). Gastrointest Endosc 2013; 77(1):29–38.

Bioengineering Lungs for Transplantation

Sarah E. Gilpin, PhD[a,b], Jonathan M. Charest, MS[a], Xi Ren, PhD[a,b], Harald C. Ott, MD[a,b],*

KEYWORDS

- Tissue engineering • Lung regeneration • Epithelium • Endothelium • Organ culture
- Bioartificial lung

KEY POINTS

- Whole lung extracellular matrix scaffolds can be created by perfusion of cadaveric organs with decellularizing detergents, providing a platform for organ regeneration.
- Lung epithelial engineering must address both the proximal airway cells that function to metabolize toxins and aid mucociliary clearance and the distal pneumocytes that facilitate gas exchange.
- Engineered pulmonary vasculature must support in vivo blood perfusion with low resistance and intact barrier function and be antithrombotic.
- Repopulating the native lung matrix with sufficient cell numbers in appropriate anatomic locations is required to enable organ function.
- The combination of mechanical, chemical, and biological stimuli can be applied to the regenerating organ during ex vivo culture in a bioreactor, allowing for testing of the maturing lung prior implantation.

INTRODUCTION

Lung transplantation remains the only curative treatment option for most advanced lung diseases.[1] Unfortunately, a substantial shortage in the availability of healthy lungs from cadaveric donors for transplantation exists. This reality is aggravated by the prevalence of cigarette smoking and associated chronic obstructive pulmonary disease, which results in an increasing demand for new therapies and donor organs.[2] Additional clinical indications for lung transplantation include idiopathic pulmonary fibrosis, cystic fibrosis, and primary pulmonary hypertension.[3] Compounding the problem, a relatively low lung utilization rate from organ donors, reported at less than 30%, contributes to long wait times for transplantation.[4] Most frequently, lung nonutilization is a result of poor organ function at the time of donation. One promising approach to improve donor lung function and transplantability is the ex vivo lung perfusion system (EVLP [XVIVO Perfusion AB,

Göteborg Sweden]).[5] This technology to recondition donor lungs and restore acceptable function criteria has resulted in an expanded donor pool and an increase in total lung transplant recipients.[6] Nevertheless, this approach does not directly address the long-term issues associated with lung transplantation, which most significantly include chronic rejection and the development of bronchiolitis obliterans syndrome.[7] As a means to overcome this immune response to allografts, tissue and organ engineering proposes to create transplantable organs by combining biologically suitable scaffolds with a patient's own cells. These implantable constructs are presented as a theoretic alternative to cadaveric donor organs for transplantation, which may ultimately eliminate the need for lifelong immunosuppression and provide long-lasting therapeutic benefits to patients in need. The challenges of scaffold production, optimal cell choice for regeneration, and the appropriate design of biomimetic culture systems are discussed.

The authors have nothing to disclose.
a Department of Surgery, Massachusetts General Hospital, Boston, MA 02114, USA; b Harvard Medical School, Boston, MA 02115, USA
* Corresponding author. Department of Surgery, Massachusetts General Hospital, Boston, MA 02114.
E-mail address: hott@mgh.harvard.edu

Thorac Surg Clin 26 (2016) 163–171
http://dx.doi.org/10.1016/j.thorsurg.2015.12.004

THE SCAFFOLD: DECELLULARIZED NATIVE EXTRACELLULAR MATRIX

In order to engineer solid organs with the biological complexity of their native counterparts and the capacity to regain appropriate physiologic functions following transplantation, the foundation on which to build is an important consideration. Much evidence has demonstrated that the process of whole organ decellularization can provide an ideal framework for regeneration. By accessing the organ's native vascular network, detergents or other recellularizing agents can be delivered in a controlled and extensive manner throughout the organ, first lysing the endogenous cellular elements and then effectively removing the resulting debris. Whole, perfusion-based lung decellularization was first reported in rodents,[8,9] validating the concept and providing an initial proof-of-concept framework for generating whole organ scaffolds. Commonly used detergents include the anionic sodium dodecyl sulfate and sodium deoxycholatedeoxycholate and the zwitterionic detergent, 3-[(3-cholamidopropyl) dimethylammonio]-1-propanesulfonate. The minimal criteria proposed to confirm adequate decellularization are less than 50 ng dsDNA retained per milligram extracellular matrix (ECM) dry weight, less than 200 bp DNA fragment length, and visible loss of nuclear material following DAPI (4′,6-diamidino-2-phenylindole) or H&E (hematoxylin and eosin) stain.[10] Deeper analysis of the resulting lung matrices generated following detergent perfusion has demonstrated preservation of the native organ architecture, supported by the retention of essential extracellular proteins.[11,12] Detailed proteomic analysis by mass spectrometry confirmed that decellularized lung matrix is predominantly composed of structural collagens, laminin, and elastin and also retains varying degrees of proteoglycans and glycoproteins.[11,13,14] Maintenance of intact structural compartmentalization has also been demonstrated for the acellular lung scaffolds, with a preserved basement membrane extending throughout the vascular network and delicate distal airspaces. The retention of these key biological elements, in the correct anatomic locations, is important to facilitate the eventual reintroduction of specialized cells types to the appropriate location. Initial biocompatibility of the scaffold in coculture with epithelial cells, endothelial cells, fibroblasts, and mesenchymal stem cells has been demonstrated.[9,15]

To translate the decellularization procedure to a clinically relevant size, the initial methodologies have been successfully up-scaled to porcine, macaque, and human donor lungs.[16,17] The ease of scaling this procedure to human-size organs provides an advantage over other manufactured scaffolds, including those made of crosslinked polyglycolic acid, collagen, or Gelfoam (Pfizer, New York, USA) which are not ideal for large-scale organ engineering.[18–20] Validation of the decellularized large lungs scaffolds has confirmed a similar preservation of organ architecture and matrix composition, further supporting the utility of this procedure for clinical-scale bioengineering.[11] The structure of the native lung is largely determined by the complex network of matrix and connective tissue in functional mechanical units.[21] Maintaining this microarchitecture within the decellularized scaffold is required for subsequent reacquisition of essential organ biomechanics. Following cell removal and any accompanying cell-derived materials, such as glycosaminoglycans and pulmonary surfactant, the dynamic mechanics of the system are dramatically altered. Precise measurement of whole organ biomechanics using traditional pulmonary functions tests, such as compliance and resistance, is challenging when applied to an acellular scaffold.[22] Changes to the mechanical properties of decellularized lung tissue may vary depending on the detergent and decellularization approach used.[23] It is important to note that changes in local stiffness may not directly translate to alterations in global biomechanics, but may have significant effects on the cells repopulating a specific microenvironment.[24] The true consequences of lung decellularization on functional mechanics may be most appropriately assessed following recellularization and organ culture, as a critical test before implantation.

Thinking toward clinical application, the establishment of minimally acceptable criteria for a decellularized lung scaffold may be required, including ECM composition, bioburden, and immunogenicity. There are little currently reported data addressing the immune response of a recipient to decellularized lung matrix, which highlights a crucial area of required study. Another important consideration that requires further investigation is the source of donor organs. Scaffolds derived from individuals with known lung diseases, including emphysema and fibrosis, may retain biological cues that can negatively influence the behavior of reintroduced cells and recapitulate disease phenotypes.[25,26] Many questions remain regarding the effect of donor age and species when developing the optimal platform for regeneration. At minimum, the biological lung scaffold must be able to support the attachment and growth of various reintroduced cell types, without significantly altering their phenotype or inhibiting their function. Significant challenges remain concerning the optimum cells choice, the methodologies for expansion to required cell numbers, and the techniques for adequate cell delivery throughout a human-scale organ.

The delivery of specialized cell populations to their appropriate biological location, coupled with ex vivo culture and tissue maturation, provides a framework to regenerate functional lungs for human therapeutic benefit (**Fig. 1**).

AIRWAY: REGENERATING LUNG EPITHELIUM

The successful regeneration of functional lung tissue through recellularization of the native scaffold will require the targeted replacement of specialized lung epithelial cell types in distinct anatomic locations. The human lung epithelium comprises many distinctive cell types,[27] which can be loosely categorized into proximal and distal phenotypes each with unique and important functions. The acellular scaffold structure allows for the direct delivery of large cell numbers through the main airways, which can easily reach to the distal airspaces. The aim of re-establishing an organized epithelium with functional cell biology and physiology presents many questions and challenges.

The proximal airways are lined with pseudostratified columnar epithelium that is mainly composed of secretory club cells, ciliated cells,

goblet cells, and the anchoring basal cell population.[28] The total surface area from the trachea to bronchioles is estimated at approximately 2500 cm^2 in human lungs and estimated to contain 10.5×10^9 cells.[29] When considering the goal of reconstituting a full airway epithelium on decellularized lung scaffolds, this fact highlights the need for an easily expandable and robust cell source. The cell source must also contain, or be capable of generating, several distinct airway epithelial lineages. Basal cells are a relatively undifferentiated population that comprise approximately 30% of the human airways[29] and that have been demonstrated to have stem cell properties.[30] In animal models of lung injury, basal cells become highly proliferative and can differentiate to re-establish both secretory and ciliated epithelium. In human bronchi, basal cells have a large surface area in contact with the basement membrane $(51.3 \pm 4.6 \ \mu m^2/cell)^{[29]}$ and express abundant cytoskeletal, junctional, and adhesive proteins.[31] Together, these attributes make basal cells an attractive option for airway engineering on decellularized scaffolds. Recapitulating the essential functions of the airway epithelium, including mucous production and mucociliary transport to clear airborne debris, immune system regulation, and control of airway fluid balance, is a challenging requirement for a regenerated tissue.

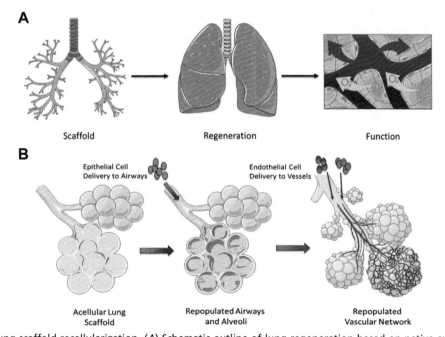

Fig. 1. Lung scaffold recellularization. (*A*) Schematic outline of lung regeneration based on native extracellular matrices. (*B*) Delivery of epithelial cells to the decellularized airways, combined with delivery of endothelial cell populations to the vascular network will allow for repopulation and regeneration of the essential gas exchange structures. (*Courtesy of* Servier Medical Arts, Neuilly-sur-Seine, France.)

Minimal essential criteria may be required for initial construct development, which would evolve as tissue engineering and cell biology coalesce.

The most basic required function of an implantable engineered lung would be gas exchange to support life. In healthy lungs, this occurs by passive diffusion, as several liters of air are bidirectionally transferred from the external environment to the alveolar space every minute. The total alveolar surface area has been measured at more than 1×10^6 cm^2 in human lungs and comprise type 1 and type 2 pneumocytes. It is estimated that there are 18 times more alveolar cells than bronchial epithelial cells, totaling almost 2×10^{11} pneumocytes.[29] Nevertheless, each alveolar structure contains a balance of type 1 and type 2 pneumocytes, with the average human alveolus being covered by 40 type I and 67 type II cells.[27] Further complexity is found in cell size and surface area, as it has been reported that type I cells comprise approximately 8% of the cells in the lung, but cover more than 95% of the surface area because of their thin, elongated shape.[27] It is this morphology that facilitates gas exchange across the interface of the alveolar type 1 cells and the pulmonary capillary endothelial cells. Type 1 cells are also critical for ion and fluid transport.[32] When considering approaches to engineer and regenerate the alveolar structure, preserving cell arrangement and morphology will be critical to maintaining efficient gas diffusion. Type 2 pneumocytes represent approximately 14% of all lung cells, but cover less than 5% of the epithelial surface.[27] In vivo, type 2 pneumocytes synthesize, secrete, and recycle surfactant components, transport ions, and participate in lung immune responses.[33] Type 2 pneumocytes also function as the progenitor cell for type 1 pneumocytes, aiding in repair after injury and maintaining tissue homeostasis.[33] The isolation and primary culture of type 1 and type 2 pneumocytes in vitro are technically challenging. Early senescence and phenotypic drift are often observed in isolated cultures.[34] Generating sufficient alveolar cell numbers through primary tissue isolation will not likely be an effective approach for large-scale lung epithelial engineering. Alternate sources of alveolar cell lineage for recellularization may include the differentiation of primary basal cells toward distal lung phenotypes,[35] or the directed differentiation of pluripotent stem cells.[36] Considering the complexity and specialized nature of the lung epithelium, many engineering and cell biology challenges clearly remain toward the aim of whole lung regeneration.

VASCULATURE: REGENERATING THE LUNG ENDOTHELIUM

The regeneration of functional pulmonary vasculature must, at minimum, allow for physiologic blood perfusion following implantation. The preservation of essential anatomic features in the decellularized lung scaffold allows for direct delivery of endothelial cells through the vascular outlets in order to reconstruct the vasculature network. The native matrix architecture also facilitates direct anastomosis of the graft to the recipient after regeneration.

Initial studies of lung bioengineering have mainly used primary rodent and human endothelial cells to recellularize the vascular compartment. A human lung is estimated to contain approximately 75×10^9 endothelial cells.[37,38] With the goal of regenerating pulmonary vasculature of human-sized lungs for clinical use, the source of endothelial cells must be scalable and patient-derived. Autologous endothelial progenitor cells and endothelial cells derived from human-induced pluripotent stem cells (hiPSCs) are promising candidates. However, endothelial progenitor cells isolated from adult peripheral blood can only be expanded for 20 to 30 population doublings during in vitro expansion, comparing to more than 100 doublings from cord blood progenitors.[39] As an alternative to endothelial progenitors isolated from autologous blood, endothelial colony-forming cells can be generated through differentiation of hiPSCs and exhibit expansion potential similar to cord blood-derived endothelial progenitors.[40] Endothelial cells derived from cord blood and peripheral blood endothelial progenitor cells[41,42] and those differentiated from hiPSCs[43] are capable of forming perfusable vascular networks in 3-dimensional matrices following in vivo subcutaneous implantation.

Morphologically, capillaries from various organs exhibit distinct differences. For example, capillaries in the lung, brain, and heart are continuous and nonfenestrated; capillaries from kidney glomeruli are continuous but fenestrated, and capillaries from the liver are discontinuous.[44] Consistent with the morphologic heterogeneity, RNA profiling indicated organ/tissue-specific molecular signatures across capillary endothelial cells.[45] In addition to heterogeneity between organs, endothelial cells within an organ also differ according to their location in the vascular tree; this includes large-diameter and smooth muscle-rich arteries, large-diameter veins with much less smooth muscle compared with arteries, and capillaries that are largely devoid of smooth muscle cells but associated with pericytes. During development, the proximal pulmonary arteries and veins are derived from cardiac mesoderm; however, the distal pulmonary capillaries are derived from a separate distinct mesodermal population.[46] The specification of pulmonary capillaries, but not proximal pulmonary endothelium, depends on the codevelopment of lung epithelium.[46] Moreover, the molecular differences between arterial and venous endothelial cells are established very early in vascular specification,[47] highlighting their fundamental differences. In light of this endothelial heterogeneity, the use of pulmonary-specific endothelial cells and the recapitulation of the spatial difference inside the pulmonary vascular tree need to be considered in tissue engineering approaches.

For pulmonary vascular engineering, endothelial cells are not the only required cell type. Perivascular cells and smooth muscle cells are also essential populations. Three-dimensional gel matrix models have demonstrated that mesenchymal support cells play a critical role in stabilizing the vascular networks in vivo.[43,48] Engineering pulmonary arteries with functional smooth muscle cells may be an additional requirement to achieve reactive vasculature that responds to physiologic clues and appropriately regulate pulmonary blood flow to enable ventilation-perfusion matching.

Reconstitution of pulmonary vascular functions in acellular lung scaffolds should allow for blood perfusion with low resistance, should prevent edema and leakage of blood components into the airway compartment,[8,9] and should be antithrombotic.[8] To attain these functional endpoints, the acellular pulmonary vascular bed needs to be repopulated with viable and functional endothelial cells and achieve robust endothelial coverage throughout the lung.

Immediately following endothelial cell delivery, the lung vascular bed is filled with a disorganized cell mixture. Massive vascular remodeling must occur in order to transition cells toward a flattened morphology, to achieve basement membrane coverage and perfusable vascular lumens. This transition mimics the process of endothelial remodeling during vascular development.[49,50] Stimulation with angiogenic growth factors can promote vascular remodeling in 3-dimensional gel matrices, leading to vascular lumen formation and the establishment of apical-basal polarity.[51–53] To date, the culture of bioengineered lungs has primarily used conventional endothelial cell culture medium.[8,9] Optimization of growth media components, and the subsequent characterization of vascular lumen development at both the macrovascular and microvascular scale, remains an important area of investigation in lung vascular engineering. Functional assessment of the regenerating lung during ex vivo culture, including pulmonary vascular perfusability, vascular resistance, and vascular leakage and barrier function, is also an essential determinant of graft maturity and readiness for implantation.

FROM CELL-SEEDED CONSTRUCTS TO FUNCTIONAL TISSUE: BIOREACTORS AND WHOLE ORGAN CULTURE

To properly develop ex vivo methodologies for whole organ culture and regeneration, one must consider the native biological context. Basic lung function in vivo depends on specific mechanical events that facilitate the exchange of gases between the perfusing blood and inspired air. These parameters have direct effects on the organ, tissue, cellular, and subcellular scales. Therefore, recapitulating these biomimetic events ex vivo is a critical component of lung bioengineering. The 2 primary events involved in lung function are blood perfusion through the vasculature and ventilation of the airways. Through organ culture in a specialized bioreactor, discrete biomimetic cues can be directly applied and manipulated in order to positively influence lung regeneration.

In vivo lung perfusion is facilitated by the right heart, which pumps deoxygenated blood into the pulmonary artery (PA). The mechanical event of pumping discrete stroke volumes into the lung transfers repetitive forces to the lung vasculature. For example, the oscillation of pressure within the PA directly translates into cyclic circumferential stretching of vessel walls. This force is seen directly by the ECM and the cells that reside in the vessel walls, including endothelial and smooth muscle cells. These cell types are particularly sensitive to such stimuli.[54] In addition, the delivery of shear stress to the endothelial cells lining the vessel walls can also influence endothelial cell alignment, behavior, and homeostasis.[54,55] Furthermore, perfusion facilitates nutrient delivery and waste removal through physical transport phenomena while maintaining the desired chemical gradients.

Lung ventilation in vivo is driven by a continuous volume change facilitated by expansion and relaxation of the chest cavity. During inspiration, an increase in chest cavity volume forces the lungs to expand with a corresponding drop in alveolar and airway pressures, causing air to flow into the lungs. The reverse happens during expiration and air is driven out of the lungs. These events translate into the cyclic stretching and relaxation of the lung parenchyma comprising cells and

ECM.[56] Cyclic stretch can induce behavioral changes in lung epithelial cells, including surfactant secretion, differentiation, and cytokine release.[57] Sufficient ventilation is further required to maintain the chemical gradients that drive O_2 delivery and CO_2 removal.

Under healthy conditions in vivo, a state of homeostasis is maintained between the cells, the ECM, and their environment. Changes in the cellular microenvironment via the ECM can directly influence cellular behavior. Cells translate mechanical cues from their microenvironment into biological signals through mechanotransduction, which directly influences cell morphology, migration, and gene expression.[58,59] Chemical gradients also influence a variety of cell behaviors.[60–62] These factors are particularly relevant when engineering a lung based on native ECM scaffolds.[63]

An emerging challenge in lung bioengineering is determining the most effective means to introduce these stimuli to regenerating lung. Various bioreactors[8,9,64–67] have been developed to fill this niche, giving the researcher significant control over the biological, mechanical, and chemical environment of the cultured organ, with most designs incorporating mechanisms for both perfusion and ventilation. The primary determinant of bioreactor design is the scale of the graft being regenerated, because the perfusion-ventilation effects to be delivered must be matched to the corresponding physiology. For example, the cardiac output of a rat is on the order of 10 to 20 mL/min,[68] while human and porcine cardiac outputs are several liters per minute. Total lung capacity also differs from approximately 10 mL in rats to 5 L in human.[29] Thus, bioreactor design should aim to match normal physiology of the organism.

Secondary determinants of bioreactor design include the perfusion and ventilation mechanisms. Perfusion of the scaffold can be applied in different modes: constant flow rate, constant pressure, or oscillatory flow rate/pressure. The more complex implementations of these modes can allow for greater control over flow parameters by using computer-controlled pumps coupled with pressure sensors and flow dampeners. Monitoring and recording of arterial and venous pressures can also be incorporated into the design.

Ventilation can be introduced using either positive- or negative-pressure mechanisms. Both approaches generate an oscillating pressure gradient between the airways and exterior of the scaffold that drives inspiration and expiration. Negative-pressure ventilation systems may use the transport of either liquid[8,65] or air[69] to generate external pressure changes. The choice of ventilation medium is an important consideration, because fluid ventilation can be used to directly deliver trophic factors to cells seeded in the airway. Especially when seeding lung scaffolds with epithelial progenitor cells of earlier developmental stages, liquid ventilation corresponding to prenatal conditions may be required to enable tissue maturation. However, this approach is not physiologic to the postnatal or adult lung. Air ventilation more closely resembles normal physiology; however, ventilation mechanics of the scaffold will likely be altered. Air ventilation can further be used to longitudinally test the gas exchange capacity of the regenerating lung in culture.

Perfusate composition is an important consideration in lung bioengineering, which has yet to be fully optimized. Most current lung bioengineering applications use traditional cell culture media as perfusates, although choosing the appropriate medium becomes complex when multiple cell types are seeded. On the other end of this spectrum, clinical EVLP uses a high colloid solution to mitigate edema that is at times supplemented with red blood cells.[6] As engineered lungs advance in size, function, and maturity, the definition of an ideal perfusate will also evolve. Generating a fully engineered lung may require a set or spectrum of perfusates that adapt to the needs of the nascent organ. Further investigation is necessary to better define these perfusates.

The combination of mechanical, chemical, and biological stimuli within an optimized bioreactor design will ultimately yield a functional graft from a reseeded decellularized scaffold (**Fig. 2**). The time points at which to introduce these stimuli, and quantitative and qualitative specifications, are yet to be defined. A potential timeline of biomimetic culture for lung regeneration (see **Fig. 2**) would involve the gradual introduction of stimuli alongside cellular repopulation and growth. Pragmatically, the inclusion of biomimetic elements in regeneration protocols provides a means to test and assess organ function during the regeneration process. Sufficient performance of the graft in these assessments can be used to establish meaningful, quantitative criteria for transplant readiness.

APPLICATION: TRANSPLANTATION OF REGENERATED LUNG CONSTRUCTS

A major aim of regenerative medicine is to develop clinically viable approaches to re-create human organs and tissues that recapitulate both the structure and the function of the native organ; this is of particular importance in the context of end-stage organ failure. Technologies such as

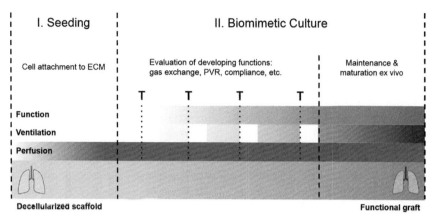

Fig. 2. Proposed timeline of biomimetic culture applied for lung regeneration from decellularized scaffold to functional graft. After an initial seeding phase, biomimetic stimuli are gradually introduced alongside testing (T) of physiologically relevant parameters. Critical tests of organ function during ex vivo regeneration include gas exchange capacity, pulmonary vascular resistance (PVR), and lung compliance. The ability to assess the maturing organ before implantation is an important consideration when designing the bioreactor system.

cardiopulmonary bypass and extracorporeal membrane oxygenation are well developed in the clinical setting, but only provide short-term solutions and are nonambulatory. Although these options provide the basic requirement of gas exchange, issues of coagulation and infection remain. Promising alternative membrane oxygenators, such as the NovaLung (Xenios AG, Heilbronn, Germany), are being developed as a bridge to transplant,[70] but the ultimate need for donor organs remains.

The goal of re-creating the complexity of the lung on a native matrix scaffold is daunting. Aiming to place each cell back in the correct location and reacquiring intricate cellular functions may be beyond the scope of the most talented cell biologist and engineers. Following reintroduction of cells to the scaffold and defined culture ex vivo, transition to an in vivo culture phase may be required to achieve full graft maturity. Blood-derived factors, as well as exogenous circulating cell populations, may be required for complete organ regeneration and reacquisition of full function. Nevertheless, accomplishing minimal functional criteria such as perfusability and gas diffusion may have immediate clinical benefit; this will likely be initially realized as a single regenerated lung or isolated lobe for implantation, possibly even as a bridging device rather than a destination treatment. Defining the functional criteria for an implantable lung construct will require controlled large animal studies and long-term evaluation.

SUMMARY

The ability to create an implantable gas exchange construct on demand, from patient-derived cells,

would have significant benefit to patients. Much work is still required to fully coalesce the fields of matrix and cell biology with tissue engineering, but promising advances have already been realized. Important questions regarding cell source, expansion, and delivery are currently being addressed, in order to ultimately achieve functional tissue formation and construct implantation.

REFERENCES

1. McCurry KR, Shearon TH, Edwards LB, et al. Lung transplantation in the United States, 1998-2007. Am J Transplant 2009;9(4 Pt 2):942–58.
2. Renteria E, Jha P, Forman D, et al. The impact of cigarette smoking on life expectancy between 1980 and 2010: a global perspective. Tob Control 2015. [Epub ahead of print].
3. Christie JD, Edwards LB, Aurora P, et al. Registry of the International Society for Heart and Lung Transplantation: twenty-fifth official adult lung and heart/lung transplantation report–2008. J Heart Lung Transplant 2008; 27(9):957–69.
4. Hornby K, Ross H, Keshavjee S, et al. Non-utilization of hearts and lungs after consent for donation: a Canadian multicentre study. Can J Anaesth 2006;53(8): 831–7.
5. Cypel M, Keshavjee S. Extending the donor pool: rehabilitation of poor organs. Thorac Surg Clin 2015;25(1):27–33.
6. Machuca TN, Cypel M. Ex vivo lung perfusion. J Thorac Dis 2014;6(8):1054–62.
7. Weigt SS, DerHovanessian A, Wallace WD, et al. Bronchiolitis obliterans syndrome: the Achilles' heel of lung transplantation. Semin Respir Crit Care Med 2013;34(3):336–51.

8. Petersen TH, Calle EA, Zhao L, et al. Tissue-engineered lungs for in vivo implantation. Science 2010;329(5991):538–41.

9. Ott HC, Clippinger B, Conrad C, et al. Regeneration and orthotopic transplantation of a bioartificial lung. Nat Med 2010;16(8):927–33.

10. Crapo PM, Gilbert TW, Badylak SF. An overview of tissue and whole organ decellularization processes. Biomaterials 2011;32(12):3233–43.

11. Gilpin SE, Guyette JP, Gonzalez G, et al. Perfusion decellularization of human and porcine lungs: bringing the matrix to clinical scale. J Heart Lung Transplant 2014;33(3):298–308.

12. Petersen TH, Calle EA, Colehour MB, et al. Matrix composition and mechanics of decellularized lung scaffolds. Cells Tissues Organs 2012;195(3): 222–31.

13. Wagner DE, Bonenfant NR, Sokocevic D, et al. Three-dimensional scaffolds of acellular human and porcine lungs for high throughput studies of lung disease and regeneration. Biomaterials 2014; 35(9):2664–79.

14. Hill RC, Calle EA, Dzieciatkowska M, et al. Quantification of extracellular matrix proteins from a rat lung scaffold to provide a molecular readout for tissue engineering. Mol Cell Proteomics 2015; 14(4):961–73.

15. Daly AB, Wallis JM, Borg ZD, et al. Initial binding and recellularization of decellularized mouse lung scaffolds with bone marrow-derived mesenchymal stromal cells. Tissue Eng Part A 2012;18(1–2):1–16.

16. Bonvillain RW, Danchuk S, Sullivan DE, et al. A nonhuman primate model of lung regeneration: detergent-mediated decellularization and initial in vitro recellularization with mesenchymal stem cells. Tissue Eng Part A 2012;18(23–24):2437–52.

17. Guyette JP, Gilpin SE, Charest JM, et al. Perfusion decellularization of whole organs. Nat Protoc 2014; 9(6):1451–68.

18. Chen P, Marsilio E, Goldstein RH, et al. Formation of lung alveolar-like structures in collagen-glycosaminoglycan scaffolds in vitro. Tissue Eng 2005;11(9–10):1436–48.

19. Mondrinos MJ, Koutzaki S, Jiwanmall E, et al. Engineering three-dimensional pulmonary tissue constructs. Tissue Eng 2006;12(4):717–28.

20. Andrade CF, Wong AP, Waddell TK, et al. Cell-based tissue engineering for lung regeneration. Am J Physiol Lung Cell Mol Physiol 2007;292(2):L510–8.

21. Suki B, Ito S, Stamenovic D, et al. Biomechanics of the lung parenchyma: critical roles of collagen and mechanical forces. J Appl Physiol (1985) 2005; 98(5):1892–9.

22. Nichols JE, Niles J, Riddle M, et al. Production and assessment of decellularized pig and human lung scaffolds. Tissue Eng Part A 2013;19(17–18): 2045–62.

23. O'Neill JD, Anfang R, Anandappa A, et al. Decellularization of human and porcine lung tissues for pulmonary tissue engineering. Ann Thorac Surg 2013;96(3):1046–55 [discussion: 1055–6].

24. Melo E, Garreta E, Luque T, et al. Effects of the decellularization method on the local stiffness of acellular lungs. Tissue Eng Part C Methods 2014; 20(5):412–22.

25. Wagner DE, Bonenfant NR, Parsons CS, et al. Comparative decellularization and recellularization of normal versus emphysematous human lungs. Biomaterials 2014;35(10):3281–97.

26. Booth AJ, Hadley R, Cornett AM, et al. Acellular normal and fibrotic human lung matrices as a culture system for in vitro investigation. Am J Respir Crit Care Med 2012;186(9):866–76.

27. Stone KC, Mercer RR, Gehr P, et al. Allometric relationships of cell numbers and size in the mammalian lung. Am J Respir Cell Mol Biol 1992;6(2):235–43.

28. Li F, He J, Wei J, et al. Diversity of epithelial stem cell types in adult lung. Stem Cells Int 2015;2015: 728307.

29. Mercer RR, Russell ML, Roggli VL, et al. Cell number and distribution in human and rat airways. Am J Respir Cell Mol Biol 1994;10(6):613–24.

30. Rock JR, Onaitis MW, Rawlins EL, et al. Basal cells as stem cells of the mouse trachea and human airway epithelium. Proc Natl Acad Sci U S A 2009; 106(31):12771–5.

31. Evans MJ, van Winkle LS, Fanucchi MV, et al. Cellular and molecular characteristics of basal cells in airway epithelium. Exp Lung Res 2001; 27(5):401–15.

32. Dobbs LG, Johnson MD. Alveolar epithelial transport in the adult lung. Respir Physiol Neurobiol 2007; 159(3):283–300.

33. Guillot L, Nathan N, Tabary O, et al. Alveolar epithelial cells: master regulators of lung homeostasis. Int J Biochem Cell Biol 2013;45(11):2568–73.

34. Gonzalez R, Yang YH, Griffin C, et al. Freshly isolated rat alveolar type I cells, type II cells, and cultured type II cells have distinct molecular phenotypes. Am J Physiol Lung Cell Mol Physiol 2005; 288(1):L179–89.

35. Vaughan AE, Brumwell AN, Xi Y, et al. Lineage-negative progenitors mobilize to regenerate lung epithelium after major injury. Nature 2015; 517(7536):621–5.

36. Huang SX, Green MD, de Carvalho AT, et al. The in vitro generation of lung and airway progenitor cells from human pluripotent stem cells. Nat Protoc 2015;10(3):413–25.

37. Crapo J, Barry B, Gehr P, et al. Cell number and cell characteristics of the normal human lung. Am Rev Respir Dis 1982;126(2):332–7.

38. Stone K, Mercer R, Freeman B, et al. Distribution of lung cell numbers and volumes between alveolar

and nonalveolar tissue. Am Rev Respir Dis 1992;
146(2):454–6.

39. Ingram DA, Mead LE, Tanaka H, et al. Identification of a novel hierarchy of endothelial progenitor cells using human peripheral and umbilical cord blood. Blood 2004;104(9):2752–60.

40. Prasain N, Lee MR, Vemula S, et al. Differentiation of human pluripotent stem cells to cells similar to cord-blood endothelial colony-forming cells. Nat Biotechnol 2014;32(11):1151–7.

41. Melero-Martin JM, De Obaldia ME, Kang S-Y, et al. Engineering robust and functional vascular networks in vivo with human adult and cord blood-derived progenitor cells. Circ Res 2008;103(2):194–202.

42. Au P, Daheron LM, Duda DG, et al. Differential in vivo potential of endothelial progenitor cells from human umbilical cord blood and adult peripheral blood to form functional long-lasting vessels. Blood 2008; 111(3):1302–5.

43. Samuel R, Daheron L, Liao S, et al. Generation of functionally competent and durable engineered blood vessels from human induced pluripotent stem cells. Proc Natl Acad Sci U S A 2013; 110(31):12774–9.

44. Aird WC. Phenotypic heterogeneity of the endothelium. Circ Res 2007;100(2):174–90.

45. Nolan DJ, Ginsberg M, Israely E, et al. Molecular signatures of tissue-specific microvascular endothelial cell heterogeneity in organ maintenance and regeneration. Dev Cell 2013;26(2):204–19.

46. Peng T, Tian Y, Boogerd CJ, et al. Coordination of heart and lung co-development by a multipotent cardiopulmonary progenitor. Nature 2013;500(7464): 589–92.

47. Swift MR, Weinstein BM. Arterial-venous specification during development. Circ Res 2009;104(5): 576–88.

48. Au P, Tam J, Fukumura D, et al. Bone marrow-derived mesenchymal stem cells facilitate engineering of long-lasting functional vasculature. Blood 2008;111(9):4551–8.

49. Herbert SP, Stainier DY. Molecular control of endothelial cell behaviour during blood vessel morphogenesis. Nat Rev Mol Cell Biol 2011;12(9):551–64.

50. Strilić B, Kučera T, Eglinger J, et al. The molecular basis of vascular lumen formation in the developing mouse aorta. Dev Cell 2009;17(4):505–15.

51. Bayless KJ, Salazar R, Davis GE. RGD-dependent vacuolation and lumen formation observed during endothelial cell morphogenesis in three-dimensional fibrin matrices involves the αvβ3 and α5β1 integrins. Am J Pathol 2000;156(5):1673–83.

52. Bayless KJ, Davis GE. The Cdc42 and Rac1 GTPases are required for capillary lumen formation in three-dimensional extracellular matrices. J Cell Sci 2002;115(6):1123–36.

53. Lampugnani MG, Orsenigo F, Rudini N, et al. CCM1 regulates vascular-lumen organization by inducing endothelial polarity. J Cell Sci 2010; 123(7):1073–80.

54. Chien S. Mechanotransduction and endothelial cell homeostasis: the wisdom of the cell. Am J Physiol Heart Circ Physiol 2007;292(3):H1209–24.

55. Carey SP, Charest JM, Reinhart-King CA. Forces during cell adhesion and spreading: implications for cellular homeostasis. In: Gefen A, editor. Cellular and biomolecular mechanics and mechanobiology. Berlin: Springer Berlin Heidelberg; 2011. p 29–60.

56. Suki D, Stamenovic D, Hubmayr R. Lung parenchymal mechanics. Compr Physiol 2011;1(3): 1317–51.

57. Waters CM, Roan E, Navajas D. Mechanobiology in lung epithelial cells: measurements, perturbations, and responses. Compr Physiol 2012;2(1): 1–29.

58. Ingber DE. Cellular mechanotransduction: putting all the pieces together again. FASEB J 2006;20(7): 811–27.

59. Wozniak MA, Chen CS. Mechanotransduction in development: a growing role for contractility. Nat Rev Mol Cell Biol 2009;10(1):34–43.

60. Crick F. Diffusion in embryogenesis. Nature 1970; 225(5231):420–2.

61. Tabata T. Genetics of morphogen gradients. Nat Rev Genet 2001;2(8):620–30.

62. Nelson CM. Geometric control of tissue morphogenesis. Biochim Biophys Acta 2009;1793(5):903–10.

63. Balestrini JL, Niklason LE. Extracellular matrix as a driver for lung regeneration. Ann Biomed Eng 2015;43(3):568–76.

64. Price AP, England KA, Matson AM, et al. Development of a decellularized lung bioreactor system for bioengineering the lung: the matrix reloaded. Tissue Eng Part A 2010;16(8):2581–91.

65. Petersen TH, Calle EA, Colehour MB, et al. Bioreactor for the long-term culture of lung tissue. Cell Transplant 2011;20(7):1117–26.

66. Song JJ, Kim SS, Liu Z, et al. Enhanced in vivo function of bioartificial lungs in rats. Ann Thorac Surg 2011;92(3):998–1005 [discussion: 10056].

67. Bonvillain RW, Scarritt ME, Pashos NC, et al. Nonhuman primate lung decellularization and recellularization using a specialized large-organ bioreactor. J Vis Exp 2013;(82):e50825.

68. Kohn DF, Clifford CB. Biology and diseases of rats. San Diego (CA): Academic Press; 2002.

69. Charest JM, Okamoto T, Kitano K, et al. Design and validation of a clinical-scale bioreactor for long-term isolated lung culture. Biomaterials 2015;52:79–87.

70. Camboni D, Philipp A, Arlt M, et al. First experience with a paracorporeal artificial lung in humans. ASAIO J 2009;55(3):304–6.

Endoscopic Resection and Ablation for Early-Stage Esophageal Cancer

Stephanie Worrell, MD, Steven R. DeMeester, MD*

KEYWORDS

- Esophageal cancer • Barrett's esophagus • Endoscopic resection • Ablation
- Esophageal adenocarcinoma

KEY POINTS

- Endoscopic resection for esophageal adenocarcinoma limited to the mucosa has similar oncologic outcomes to those of esophagectomy.
- Endoscopic resection allows for pathologic staging of the depth of tumor invasion.
- After endoscopic therapy, careful surveillance is critical to prevent recurrence or progression of disease.

INTRODUCTION
Nature of the Problem

Esophageal cancer is the 8th leading cause of cancer death in men worldwide.[1] Overall, squamous cell is the most common histology, but in most Western countries, adenocarcinoma has become far more common.[2] Surveillance programs for Barrett's esophagus, the precursor for adenocarcinoma, led to an increase in the identification of high-grade dysplasia and superficial esophageal adenocarcinoma. Traditional therapy has been an esophagectomy, but the reduced morbidity, similar oncologic outcome, and ability to preserve the esophagus with endoscopic therapy led to a paradigm shift in the treatment of these patients.[3–5] The pillars of endoscopic therapy are endoscopic resection and mucosal ablation. Endoscopic resection (ER) is mandatory for nodules or lesions in the esophagus, because if these are malignant, ablative therapies may not treat the full depth of the disease and do not provide a specimen to allow pathologic determination of the T stage of the disease. In addition to allowing pathologic assessment of the depth of tumor invasion, ER also allows evaluation of features associated with a higher risk for lymph node metastases including lymphovascular invasion and tumor differentiation. In flat, non-nodular Barrett's esophagus, ablation therapies can be used to eradicate the diseased mucosa and is preferred with long-segment Barrett's to minimize the risk of stricture. Similar concepts apply to squamous dysplasia or cancer.

Patient Selection

Endotherapy and esophagectomy are similarly effective cancer therapies for patients with HGD or intramucosal cancer.[4,5] It would be inappropriate to proceed with either therapy without informing a patient about the benefits and drawbacks of both options. There are no absolute exclusion criteria for endotherapy, although esophagectomy might be more appropriate in selected individuals, including those with poor esophageal body function; severe, uncontrollable reflux symptoms; dysphagia; or frequent aspiration. Ideal candidates for endotherapy are those with short lengths of Barrett's, normal esophageal motility, and no esophagitis, stricture, or large hiatal hernia.

Department of Surgery, Keck School of Medicine, The University of Southern California, Los Angeles, CA, USA
* Corresponding author. Department of Surgery, 1510 San Pablo Street, Suite 514, Los Angeles, CA 90033.
E-mail address: sdemeester@surgery.usc.edu

Thorac Surg Clin 26 (2016) 173–176
http://dx.doi.org/10.1016/j.thorsurg.2015.12.005
1547-4127/16/$ – see front matter © 2016 Elsevier Inc. All rights reserved.

Preprocedure Planning

When endoscopic biopsies show HGD or adeno-carcinoma, the slides should be reviewed by another experienced pathologist. A repeat endoscopy with biopsies from all suspicious areas and then from 4 quadrants every 1 to 2 cm throughout the length of the columnar segment should be performed if not done at the original endoscopy.[6,7] The mucosa should be carefully examined using high-definition white light and narrow band imaging or similar electronic enhancement. Confirmed HGD or adenocarcinoma should prompt intervention in nearly all patients.

A visible abnormality or nodule must be excised by ER, as even a flat or minimally raised lesion can harbor cancer invasive beyond the mucosa. The goal of ER is to excise the full thickness of the mucosa and submucosa to allow histologic determination of the depth of invasion. There is no maximum tumor size for ER, but lesions ≥2 cm are more likely to have invaded into the submucosa and have lymph node metastases.[8]

Procedure for Endoscopic Resection

The initial technique for ER entailed the use of a cap that was fitted over the end of a standard endoscope.[9–11] Developed by Dr Inoue from Japan, these caps are available in various sizes and configurations (flat vs angled) and come with a complete kit for the procedure by Olympus. Currently, the multiband ligator by Cook (Duette; Cook Group Inc, Bloomington, IN) is used, as it is faster and easier to use and allows overlapping resections without the cookie cutter effect that occurs with use of the Inoue cap technique. In patients with squamous cell lesions, endoscopic submucosal dissection is often preferred.[12] An advantage of the band technique is that it does not require submucosal saline injection to lift the lesion. However, injection should be considered for larger lesions because failure to lift may indicate invasion into the muscularis propria. When using the band technique, the snare should be applied below the band to avoid leaving part of the specimen behind and compromising the ability to assess the full depth of invasion. When a lesion is present, every effort should be made to completely excise the lesion by applying suction when the cap is over the central-most portion of the lesion. Piecemeal resection of larger lesions is acceptable but leads to more artifact and prohibits accurate assessment of the mucosal resection margins. Although ER is most often used to excise a lesion, it can also be used to remove flat Barrett's. Short, noncircumferential tongues of columnar mucosa can be fully excised with ER, but ER of circumferential segments or those greater than 3 cm in length should be avoided to reduce the risk of stricture.[13]

Procedure for Mucosal Ablation

Ablation is the preferred option for patients with long-segment, flat Barrett's esophagus. Importantly, ablation does not produce a specimen and is not appropriate in the setting of a mucosal irregularity or nodule. Radiofrequency ablation is currently preferred in most patients given the proven clinical efficacy in Barrett's esophagus, but increasingly other options including cryoablation are used in these patients.[14] Most experience with ablation is in patients with dysplastic Barrett's, but ablation has also shown efficacy for squamous dysplasia.[15] Typically, ablation should not be done in the same setting as ER because of the risk of perforation, but if there is sufficient Barrett's tissue separate from the ER site, simultaneous ablation can be performed. Multiple radiofrequency ablation devices are available to allow circumferential or focal ablation of the abnormal mucosa.

Potential Complications and Postoperative Instructions

The biggest concern with endoscopic therapy is esophageal perforation. There is almost no risk of perforation with ablation, and only a very low risk with ER.[16] Postprocedure bleeding has been reported after ER but is more common after resection of gastric compared with esophageal lesions. Strictures can occur with ablation or ER and are more common with longer lengths of treated mucosa, particularly when circumferential. After endotherapy, patients are advised to take full liquids for 48 hours and then soft foods for another 48 hours to allow mucosal healing to begin. Follow-up endoscopy with biopsy or retreatment is scheduled for 8 weeks from the prior procedure.

CLINICAL RESULTS

Endotherapy for superficial adenocarcinoma is becoming common practice and is supported by reports of excellent long-term survival. Pech and colleagues evaluated the long-term outcomes and safety of endoscopic therapy for intramucosal adenocarcinoma in 1000 patients. Complete remission was achieved in 96.3% of patients with a 5-year overall survival of 91.5%. There were only 2 tumor-related deaths in the series. The recurrence rate was 14.5% at a median of 26.5 months. After recurrence, repeat endoscopic therapy was successful in 82% of patients. Only

Table 1
Clinical outcomes with endotherapy and esophagectomy for high-grade dysplasia and early esophageal adenocarcinoma

	Pech et al,[17] 2011	Zehetner et al,[4] 2011	Prasad et al,[5] 2009
Endotherapy	n = 76	n = 40	n = 132
Esophagectomy	n = 38	n = 61	n = 46
Follow-up			
Endotherapy	4.1 y (median)	17 mo (median)	464.4 (person-years)
Esophagectomy	3.7 y (median)	34 mo (median)	243.8 (person-years)
Remission/R0 resection			
Endotherapy	98.7% (75/76)	NA	94% (124/132)[a]
Esophagectomy	100%	NA	NR
Overall survival			
Endotherapy	89% (5 y)	94% (3 y)	83% (5 y)
Esophagectomy	93% (5 y)	94% (3 y)	95% (5 y)
Recurrence			
Endotherapy	6.6% (5/76)	20% (8/40)	12% (16/132)
Esophagectomy	0%	0%	(1/46)
Complications			
Endotherapy	17% (13/76)	0	13% (18/132)
Esophagectomy	32%	39% (24/61)	34% (17/46)
Cancer-free survival			
Endotherapy	91% (5 y)	100% (5 y)	80% (5 y)
Esophagectomy	100% (5 y)	88% (5 y)	97% (5 y)

Abbreviation: NA, not available.
[a] No evidence of carcinoma on 2 successive surveillance endoscopies.

0.04% of patients went on to require esophageal resection.[3] These results are comparable to the long-term survival seen with esophagectomy for patients with a similar stage of disease (**Table 1**).

SUMMARY

ER with ablation has become the preferred therapy for most patients with high-grade dysplasia or esophageal cancer. Oncologic outcomes are similar to those of esophagectomy with fewer complications. ER allows pathologic staging of superficial lesions and is a critical first step in the evaluation of these patients. Mucosal ablation techniques allow treatment of long segments of mucosal disease with less risk of stricture. Careful follow-up is necessary to address recurrent mucosal disease and prevent long-term failure of an endoscopic approach in these patients.

REFERENCES

1. American Cancer Society. Global cancer facts and figures 2nd edition. Atlanta (GA): American Cancer Society; 2011.

2. Lepage C, Drouillard A, Jouve JL, et al. Epidemiology and risk factors for oesophageal adenocarcinoma. Dig Liver Dis 2013;45:625–9.

3. Pech O, May A, Manner H, et al. Long-term efficacy and safety of endoscopic resection for patients with mucosal adenocarcinoma of the esophagus. Gastroenterology 2014;146:652–60.

4. Zehetner J, DeMeester SR, Hagen JA, et al. Endoscopic resection and ablation versus esophagectomy for high-grade dysplasia and intramucosal adenocarcinoma. J Thorac Cardiovasc Surg 2011;141(1):39–47.

5. Prasad GA, Wigle DA, Buttar NS, et al. Endoscopic and surgical treatment of mucosal (T1a) esophageal adenocarcinoma in barrett's esophagus. Gastrenterology 2009;137(3):1–18.

6. Levine DS, Haggitt RC, Blount PL, et al. An endoscopic biopsy protocol can differentiate high-grade dysplasia from early adenocarcinoma in Barrett's esophagus. Gastroenterology 1993;105:40–50.

7. Reid BJ, Blount PL, Feng Z, et al. Optimizing endoscopic biopsy detection of early cancers in barrett's high-grade dysplasia. Am J Gastroenterol 2000;95:3089–96.

8. Eloubeidi MA, Desmond R, Arguedas MR, et al. Prognostic factors for the survival of patients with

esophageal carcinoma in the US: the importance of tumor length and lymph node status. Cancer 2002; 95(7):1434–43.

9. Inoue H, Kawano T, Tani M, et al. Endoscopic mucosal resection using a cap: techniques for use and preventing perforation. Can J Gastroenterol 1999;13(6):477–80.

10. Inoue H, Endo M. Endoscopic mucosal resection using a transparent tube. Surg Endosc 1990;4:198–201.

11. Inoue H, Endo M, Takeshita K, et al. Endoscopic resection of early-stage esophageal cancer. Surg Endosc 1991;5:59–62.

12. Fujishiro M, Yahagi N, Kakushima N, et al. Endoscopic submucosal dissection of esophageal squamous cell neoplasms. Clin Gastroenterol Hepatol 2006;4:688–94.

13. Qumseya B, Panossian AM, Rizk C, et al. Predictors of esophageal stricture formation post endoscopic mucosal resection. Clin Endosc 2014;47(2):155–61.

14. Shaheen NJ, Sharma P, Overholy BF, et al. Radiofrequency ablation in barrett's esophagus with dysplasia. N Engl J Med 2009;360:2277–88.

15. National Institute for Health and Care Excellence. Endoscopic radiofrequency ablation for squamous dysplasia of the oesophagus. 2014. Available at: guidance.nice.org.uk/pg497.

16. Sato H, Inoue H, Ikeda H, et al. Clinical experience of esophageal perforation occurring with endoscopic submucosal dissection. Dis Esophagus 2013;27(7):617–22.

17. Pech O, Bollschweiler E, Manner H, et al. Comparison between endoscopic and surgical resection of mucosal esophageal adenocarcinoma in Barrett's esophagus at two high-volume center. Ann Surg 2011;254(1): 67–72.

Novel Technologies in Endoscopic Lung Volume Reduction

Daniela Gompelmann, MD, Felix J.F. Herth, PhD*

KEYWORDS

- Emphysema • COPD • Interventional bronchoscopy • Endoscopic lung volume reduction

KEY POINTS

- Endoscopic lung volume reduction (ELVR) presents an effective therapy in patients with advanced emphysema characterized by a forced expiratory volume in one second less than 45% to 50% and a residual volume greater than 150%, preferably greater than 200%.
- Valve therapy is a reversible blocking technique that leads to lobar atelectasis in case of low collateral ventilation and lobar occlusion.
- The partial irreversible lung volume reduction coil implantation and irreversible bronchoscopic thermal vapor ablation are effective treatment approaches independent of collateral ventilation.
- Precise patient selection with respect to pulmonary function test, emphysema distribution, and collateral ventilation are prerequisites for a successful use of the various ELVR techniques.
- The idea of the targeted lung denervation, whose safety and feasibility was confirmed in the pilot trial, is to lead to sustainable bronchodilation by ablation of parasympathetic pulmonary nerves. Further trials evaluating efficacy are warranted.
- To date, there are only a few randomized controlled trials for bronchoscopic therapy in patients with chronic obstructive pulmonary disease, so the various techniques should be performed within clinical trials or registry studies.

Chronic obstructive pulmonary disease (COPD) is one of the most common respiratory diseases worldwide with an increasing morbidity and mortality. In 1990, COPD was ranked sixth as cause of death, but is estimated to become the third leading cause of death in 2020.[1,2] The reason for increased mortality is mainly the expanding epidemic of smoking. Predominant symptoms of COPD include productive cough, shortness of breath, and subsequent limited exercise tolerance due to chronic bronchitis, irreversible bronchoconstriction, and emphysematous destruction of lung parenchyma.

Smoking cessation, pharmacologic therapy, consequent exercise training, and pulmonary rehabilitation are the most important therapeutic options that reduce symptoms and improve exercise capacity.

Long-term oxygen therapy is required in patients with chronic respiratory failure and ventilatory support is indicated in patients with significant hypercapnia and related clinical signs. However, so far, there is no curative therapeutic approach. In addition, lung transplantation, which should be discussed in appropriately selected patients with COPD, is associated with a limited long-term prognosis and thus is often considered as palliative treatment approach. Another surgical therapeutic option in patients with severe emphysema is the lung volume reduction surgery (LVRS) that was introduced by Brantigan and colleagues[3] in the 1950s, but was abandoned due to high mortality and morbidity. It was only in the 1990s that Cooper and colleagues[4] reintroduced this surgical approach that aims at the

Conflict of Interest: Lecture and travel fees from Pulmonx (D. Gompelmann); Consultant and lecture fee from Pulmonx, PneumRx, Uptake, Olypmus (F.J.F. Herth).
Pneumology and Critical Care Medicine, Thoraxklinik at University of Heidelberg, Röntgenstr. 1, Heidelberg 69126, Germany
* Corresponding author.
E-mail address: felix.herth@med.uni-heidelberg.de

reduction of hyperinflation and thus optimizes the respiratory mechanics leading to decreased breathlessness and increased exercise capacity. As lung hyperinflation is an independent predictor for all-cause mortality in patients with COPD, minimizing hyperinflation plays an important role in patients with severe COPD.[5] However, LVRS confers a survival advantage over medical therapy in only a precise selected group of patients with emphysema. Particularly patients with predominantly upper-lobe emphysema and low exercise capacity experience improvement of lung function and exercise tolerance and seem to have a survival benefit from LVRS. However, the 90-day mortality of LVRS with 7.9% was very high in a 2003 published randomised controlled trial; particularly patients with non-upper lobe emphysema and high exercise capacity were poor candidates for LVRS.[6] Therefore, the search for minimally invasive approaches with comparable benefits to LVRS but with less attendant risk was stimulated.

Since 2003, various techniques of endoscopic lung volume reduction (ELVR) that mimics the effect of LVRS are available extending the therapeutic spectrum for patients with severe COPD and emphysema. There are blocking and non-blocking ELVR techniques that are different in degree of reversibility, safety, and toxicity and whose application is dependent on the emphysema type and interlobar collateral ventilation. However, all these methods of ELVR are only worth considering in patients with advanced emphysema characterized by a forced expiratory volume in one second (FEV$_1$) of less than 45% to 50% of predicted and a residual volume (RV) greater than 150%, preferably greater than 200%.

Reversible implantation of one-way valves represents the blocking ELVR technique, for which there has been the greatest clinical experience worldwide. For valve therapy, which has already been introduced in 2003, comprehensive data including 4 randomized clinical trials (RCTs) are available. The currently available nonblocking techniques include the lung volume reduction coil (LVRC) implantation and the bronchoscopic thermal vapor ablation (BTVA). Another nonblocking technique, the polymeric lung volume reduction is currently not available due to lack of investors despite promising efficacy results. Furthermore, the creation of extra-anatomic airway bypasses that was mainly used in patients with predominant homogeneous emphysema is no longer performed, as the initial benefits following intervention did not persist within the course of 6 months.

Besides ELVR, which focuses on the reduction of hyperinflation, targeted lung denervation (TLD) is the most recent development in the field of bronchoscopic therapeutic options in patients with COPD. This technique simulates the effect of anticholinergic drugs and thus leads to sustainable bronchodilation.

The various bronchoscopic techniques for management of COPD and emphysema are shown in **Table 1**.

VALVE IMPLANTATION

Endoscopic valve implantation that is commercially available in European countries presents the only blocking and the only reversible ELVR technique. By placement of these one-way valves in the bronchi of the most emphysematous lung lobe, air is allowed to escape during expiration but not enter during inspiration and thus inducing a target lung volume reduction (TLVR). The maximum result is a complete lobar atelectasis. The target lobe is thereby defined on the basis of multidetector computed tomography (MDCT), including software emphysema analysis (eg, YACTA, "yet another CT analyzer") and perfusion scan. So far, 2 different types of valves are available that distinguish only in shape but act both as one-way valves (**Fig. 1**). The endobronchial valves (EBVs) (Zephyr; Pulmonx, Inc, Neuchatel, Switzerland; see **Fig. 1**; **Fig. 2**) are similar to bronchial stents made from nitinol and silicone, whereas the intrabronchial valves (IBVs) (Spiration; Olympus, Tokyo, Japan; see **Fig. 1**; **Fig. 3**) have a design like an umbrella with a nitinol skeleton covered by a polyurethane membrane. Different sizes of both valves are available, which are selected depending on the diameter of the bronchi of the target lobe. The valve implantation technique is a straightforward procedure technically that is performed by using a special flexible delivery catheter that can be inserted through a 2.8-mm or larger working channel of a standard bronchoscope.

Impact of Lobar Occlusion and Collateral Ventilation

Endoscopic valve placement is, to date, the best-studied ELVR technique. Since the first publications in 2003, various trials have been performed leading to expanded knowledge with this technique. The first RCT that is currently the largest trial is the Endobronchial Valve for Emphysema Palliation Trial, also known as VENT.[7] Sciurba and colleagues[7] compared 214 patients with emphysema who underwent valve therapy with 101 patients who received standard medical care. Patients who were treated by EBV developed an improvement of 4.3% in FEV$_1$, whereas the patients of the control group experienced a decrease of 2.5%. Similar benefits were observed

Table 1
Overview of the different endoscopic techniques available in management for chronic obstructive pulmonary disease and emphysema

Endoscopic Technique	Endoscopic Lung Volume Reduction (ELVR)			Targeted Lung Denervation (TLD)
	Valve Implantation	Lung Volume Reduction Coil (LVRC) Implantation	Bronchoscopic Thermal Vapor Ablation (BTVA)	
Primary objective	Target lobe volume reduction			Bronchodilation
Mechanism of action	Lobar atelectasis	Parenchymal compression	Local inflammatory reaction	Ablation of parasympathetic nerves
Reversibility	Reversible	Partially irreversible	Irreversible	Irreversible
Prerequisite	• FEV_1 <45–50% • RV >150% • Heterogeneous emphysema with upper or lower lobe predominance	• FEV_1 <45% • RV >175% • Heterogeneous emphysema with upper or lower lobe predominance • Homogeneous emphysema	• FEV_1 <45% • RV >150% • Heterogeneous emphysema with upper lobe predominance	Positive response (FEV_1 >15%) to spirometry to inhaled ipratropium bromide
Dependence of CV	Dependent	Independent	Independent	Independent
Predictors for success	• Low CV • Lobar occlusion • High amount of low attenuation clusters • High small vessel percent vascular volume	Not available at present. Predictive factors have to be evaluated in currently ongoing trials.	Heterogeneity index >1.2	Not available at present. Predictive factors have to be evaluated in currently ongoing trials.
Frequent complications	Pneumothorax	• Hemoptysis • Inflammatory reaction	Inflammatory reaction	• COPD exacerbation • Device-related events
Availability	Commercially available in European countries.			Under investigation, RCT ongoing

Abbreviations: COPD, chronic obstructive pulmonary disease; CV, collateral ventilation; FEV_1, forced expiratory volume in 1 second; RV, residual volume.

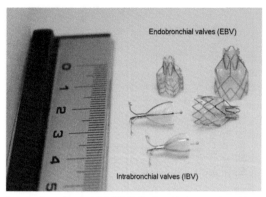

Fig. 1. Endobronchial (EBV; Zephyr, Pulmonx, Inc, Neuchatel, Schweiz) and intrabronchial (IBV; Spiration, Olympus, Tokyo, Japan) valves.

in the 6-minute walk test (6-MWT) and health-related quality of life measured by St. George's Respiratory Questionnaire (SGRQ) and modified Medical Research Council (mMRC). Overall, there was a mean between-group difference of 6.8% in the FEV_1 ($P = .005$) and of 5.8% in the 6-MWT ($P = .04$). Although these results were statistically significant, they were not clinically relevant, so that valve therapy has not been approved by the US Food and Drug Administration. However, analysis of retrospectively defined subgroups of VENT revealed predictive factors for clinical relevant improvement of outcome measures. Complete occlusion of the target lobe by the valves and complete interlobar fissure that is, defined as greater than 90% completeness of the fissure between the target and adjacent lobes on at least one axis on MDCT have impact on a

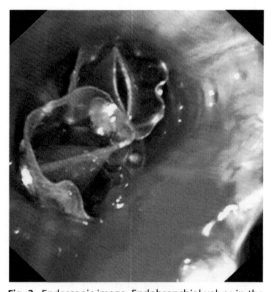

Fig. 2. Endoscopic image. Endobronchial valves in the left lower lobe.

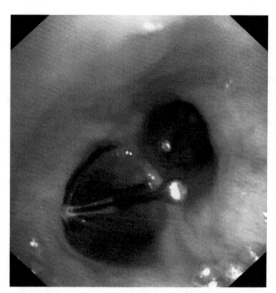

Fig. 3. Endoscopic image. Intrabronchial valves in the left upper lobe.

patient's outcome following valve placement. This hypothesis was confirmed by the European cohort of VENT (Euro-VENT).[8] At 6 months after valve therapy, patients with a complete lobar occlusion of the targeted lobe and a complete interlobar fissure in the MDCT experienced a TLVR of 80.0% ± 30% that was associated with an improvement in FEV_1 of 26% ± 24% and an increase of 6-MWT of 22% ± 38%.

The value of lobar occlusion as predictor for good outcome following valve therapy was also impressively demonstrated in the first trials using IBV. In one RCT, patients with severe emphysema who were treated by incomplete occlusion of 2 contralateral target lobes by IBV were compared with a standard medical care group.[9] The intention of incomplete occlusion was to redirect the air from emphysematous areas to healthier lung regions but to avoid the risk of pneumothorax that is higher in complete occlusion. Patients who were treated by IBV experienced an improvement of SGRQ and a volume shift from the treated to the untreated lobe but no improvement of lung function parameters or exercise test. This finding gives reason to examine the bilateral, incomplete occlusion in a direct comparison to a unilateral complete occlusion of one lobe.[10] Eleven patients with upper or lower lobe predominant emphysema underwent bilateral incomplete valve placement and were compared with 11 patients who received unilateral, but complete lobar occlusion. Results revealed an excellent outcome only in patients with unilateral treatment so that actually just a unilateral complete lobar occlusion is recommended.

Due to the knowledge that only patients with a complete interlobar fissure that seems to be a surrogate for interlobar collateral ventilation (CV) benefit from valve therapy, the interest in quantifying interlobar CV was increased. Therefore, another method than CT fissure analysis that provides evaluation of CV was developed.[11] By a catheter-based measurement using the Chartis Pulmonary Assessment System (Pulmonx, Inc, Neuchatel, Schweiz), CV can be quantified during bronchoscopy. Thereby, a dedicated catheter with a balloon at its tip is advanced in the target lobe. By inflating the balloon, the target lobe is isolated so that the airflow can be measured. A decrease of airflow during measurement indicates insignificant CV and only these "CV-negative" patients will benefit from valve therapy. The accuracy of CV assessment by using the catheter-based measurement was found to be 75%.[12] CT fissure analysis and catheter-based measurement are comparable with each other and present efficient methods to optimize patient selection before valve therapy.[13]

In a recently published RCT, known as BeLieVeR-HIFI study, only patients with intact interlobar fissures on CT were treated by complete occlusion of one target lobe by valves (n = 25) and were compared with a control group that received a sham procedure (n = 25).[14] At 3 months, FEV$_1$ increased by a mean of 24.8% (median 8.77%) in the valve group and 3.9% (median 2.88%) in the control group. Secondary measures of 6-MWT and diffusion capacity were also clinically and statistically significant. The residual volume, the COPD assessment test, and SGRQ scores improved more in the valve group but compared with the control group were not statistically significant. Regarding at radiological outcome, there was a complete lobar atelectasis in 35%, some TLVR in 30%, and no change in 35%. There were 2 deaths in the valve group within 90 days following valve placement. One of them had experienced pneumothorax after valve explantation that was performed because of cough and he progressed to respiratory failure. The other patient died due to final COPD with cor pulmonale. Overall, the results of this RCT represent the first successful sham-controlled trial of the endoscopic valve therapy in patients with severe emphysema. However, it must be mentioned that the number of patients included in that trial was much too low to demonstrate precisely safety and efficacy of valve therapy.

Further Predictors for Success of Valve Placement

Besides CT fissure integrity and lobar occlusion, further predictors for good outcome following valve

therapy were searched to optimize patient selection. In one retrospective analysis, quantitative computed tomography (QCT) parameters were examined using Apollo lung quantitative imaging software (VIDA Diagnostics, Coralville, IA).[15] QCT using VIDA Diagnostics also provides the assessment of fissure integrity that was once more confirmed to be important to reach significant TLVR following valve therapy. The accuracy for QCT patient selection based on fissure integrity was comparable to the catheter-based measurement using the Chartis Pulmonary Assessment System. Besides fissure integrity, low attenuation clusters and small vessel percent vascular volume in the target lobe were identified to be significant predictors for TLVR. Thereby, the combination of the different QCT predictors seems to be superior to fissure integrity as single predictor, but the difference did not reach the threshold for statistical significance.

Complications: Management and Prevention

Although valve implantation is a minimally invasive technique, it is also associated with complications. In VENT, the overall complication rate was 10.3% in the EBV group versus 4.6% in the standard medical care group, but the difference was not statistically significant. Within the first 3 months following valve placement, the most common adverse events were valve-related events (7.5%), COPD exacerbations (9.3%), hemoptysis (6.1%), and pneumothorax (4.2%). In recent years, however, the rate of pneumothorax increased dramatically, as low interlobar collateral ventilation is not only a predictor for good outcome following valve placement but also for the advent of pneumothorax. Actually, a pneumothorax rate of 17%[16] up to 23%[17,18] following valve placement is reported. However, as the prerequisite for the advent of lobar atelectasis and pneumothorax seems to be the same, patients who develop a pneumothorax will nevertheless benefit from valve therapy. A small number of patients with postinterventional pneumothorax experienced TLVR of 65% that was associated with great improvement in lung function parameters.[19] However, pneumothorax still remains a serious complication that requires mostly further interventions, immobilization, and prolonged hospitalization, so that strict monitoring of patients within the first 48 to 72 hours after valve implantation is crucial. Furthermore, strategies for the prevention of pneumothorax following valve placement are evaluated. In one prospective randomized trial, 40 patients underwent modified medical care including bed rest for 48 hours and cough suppression after valve placement and were compared with 32 patients who received postimplantation standard medical observation.[20] Within 3 months following valve therapy, 7.5% of the patients who underwent modified postimplantation medical care experienced pneumothorax, whereas 25% of the patients with standard medical observation developed pneumothorax. There was no significant difference in the clinical and radiological outcomes in both cohorts. Thus, it seems that bed rest for 48 hours and cough suppression after valve placement might reduce the incidence of pneumothorax. However, larger trials are needed that confirm these findings.

Summary

In summary, valve therapy presents an effective endoscopic therapy for patients with severe emphysema. With respect to selection criteria, particularly the interlobar collateral ventilation, a great outcome with improvement of lung function parameters, exercise capacity, and health-related quality of life can be achieved. Whereas valve placement is a relatively straightforward procedure technically, patient selection and the management of possible complications are the challenges.

LUNG VOLUME REDUCTION COIL IMPLANTATION

The implantation of Lung Volume Reduction Coil (LVRC; PneumRx, Inc, Mountain View, CA; **Fig. 4**) is one of the nonblocking ELVR techniques that is commercially available and in widespread use in European countries. Lung volume reduction is achieved by implantation of 10 nitinol coils in 1 target lobe that leads to compression of the lung parenchyma due to the preformed coiled shape of the LVRC. Similar to valve therapy, the target lobe is defined on the basis of MDCT and perfusion scan before coil implantation. The

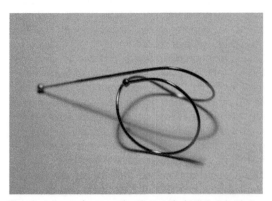

Fig. 4. Lung volume reduction coil. (LVRC; PneumRx, Inc, Mountain View, CA.)

implantation of LVRC that is available in 3 different sizes is performed bronchoscopically using a dedicated delivery system under fluoroscopic guidance. First, a low stiffness guidewire with fluoroscopic markers is inserted into the targeted airway for measuring the airway size. Afterward, the LVRC of the appropriate size is advanced in an extended form through the delivery catheter by using a forceps. By pulling the catheter back, the coil assumes its original coiled shape and can be deployed by releasing from the forceps.

The advantage of LVRC treatment compared with valve therapy is the independence from the presence or absence of interlobar collateral ventilation.[21] The disadvantage, however, is that LVRC treatment is a partial irreversible therapy.

Coils Implantation in Clinical Trials

In the 2010 published pilot trial, patients with severe heterogeneous or homogeneous emphysema were treated by 3 to 6 LVRCs in the most emphysematous lung lobe. The mean changes in efficacy endpoints were only small, but the group of patients with predominantly heterogeneous emphysema distribution experienced benefit in lung function, exercise capacity, and health-related quality of life measurements.[22] In the subsequent trial, 16 patients with heterogeneous emphysema underwent bilateral implantation of LVRCs, whereby the number of coils placed was increased up to 10 per lobe. Six months following intervention, patients experienced significant improvement of pulmonary function tests, 6-MWT, and health-related quality of life measured by SGRQ.[23] The first RCT related to LVRC implantation was the "RePneu Endobronchial Coils For the Treatment of Severe Emphysema with HyperinflaTion Trial," known as "RESET."[24] Twenty-three patients received unilateral (n = 2) or bilateral (n = 21) LVRC treatment and were compared with a standard medical care group. At 6 months, patients in the LVRC group experienced significantly greater improvement in the SGRQ (−8.11 vs 0.25 points), lung function parameters (FEV$_1$ 14.19% vs 3.57%, RV −0.51 vs 0.20 L) and 6-MWT (+51.15 vs −12.39 m) than the standard medical care group. In 2014, Deslee and colleagues[25] reported the results of the so far largest prospective LVR coil trial. In this multicenter trial, 60 patients with advanced emphysema were treated bronchoscopically by LVR coils (55 bilateral, 5 unilateral). Six months following intervention, patients experienced a significant improvement in lung function, exercise tolerance, and health-related quality of life. Longer-term analysis of the data over 1 year demonstrated a sustained response at 12 months. Post hoc CT analysis revealed that 39% of the treated patients had a homogeneous emphysema distribution. Efficacy data, demonstrated that also these patients benefited from LVRC treatment. One prospective single-arm trial confirmed that LVRC implantation seems also to provide an effective therapy for patients with predominantly homogeneous emphysema.[26] Ten patients with homogeneous emphysema who received bilateral LVRC implantation in the upper lobes experienced significant improvements for 6-MWT, lung function parameters, and SGRQ.

Long-term outcome following LVRC treatment was evaluated in another single-arm prospective trial.[27] In 22 patients who underwent coils implantation, 3-year follow-up data were available demonstrating that only the mMRC was still significantly improved compared with baseline, whereas all other clinical characteristics were not significantly changed compared with pretreatment baseline.

Complications

The most common adverse events reported in LVRC treatment include COPD exacerbation, lower respiratory tract infection, pneumonia, hemoptysis, and pneumothorax.[24,25] In one retrospective analysis, minor and major complications were precisely documented.[28] In a total of 49 LVRC procedures, a complication rate of 57% was observed. The most frequent adverse event was self-limited hemoptysis (20%). In 6% of the patients, serious hemorrhage occurred with the requirement of lobectomy in 2%. Respiratory tract infection with the need for oral (12%) or intravenous (12%) antibiotic therapy and pneumothorax (6%) that requires surgical treatment due to lung perforation by coils (4%) were reported.

Summary

In conclusion, LVRC implantation is an effective therapy in patients with advanced emphysema independent of CV. However, it must be considered that LVRC treatment is partially irreversible, so that patient selection is of great importance and predictors for good outcome following LVRC therapy have to be evaluated. Although LVRC treatment is a frequently used technique, there is actually only one RCT demonstrating the efficacy of LVRC therapy. The results of a prospective, multicenter, randomized, controlled study comparing outcomes between the LVRC and Control Groups (RENEW trial) are expected in 2016.

BRONCHOSCOPIC THERMAL VAPOR ABLATION

Bronchoscopic Thermal Vapor Ablation (BTVA, Uptake Medical Corporation, Seattle, WA) is another nonblocking ELVR technique that leads to lung volume reduction by inducing a local inflammatory reaction in the most emphysematous lung segments by instillation of heated water vapor.

Before intervention, the target airway for procedure as well as the vapor dose that depends on the density and volume of the target lung tissue is identified on the basis of the patient's MDCT by using a special software. For performing BTVA, a dedicated InterVapor catheter is advanced into the target segment. A balloon at the distal tip of this catheter is inflated, so that the target airway is isolated. Afterward, the 75°C heated water vapor is delivered. Thereafter, the balloon is deflated and the vapor treatment is repeated in the next target airway, whereby the time between 2 vapor treatments should be 3 minutes or more. The heated water vapor leads to inflammatory reaction that results in fibrosis and scarring and thus to a lung volume reduction 8 to 12 weeks after intervention.

Similar to the nonblocking LVRC treatment, BTVA is independent of collateral ventilation[29] and represents an irreversible technique. In contrast to LVRC therapy that is performed in upper or lower lobe predominant emphysema, BTVA is so far used only in patients with upper lobe predominant emphysema. To date, BTVA is the only technique in which no implants are left. Moreover, BTVA allows a targeted therapy of emphysematous lung segments and thus BTVA has the potential to manage intralobar heterogeneous upper lobe predominant emphysema.

So far, there is only one RCT related to BTVA, known as "Step-Up trial," which was completed in late 2014. Given the results of this RCT, the InterVapor System received a CE (Conformité Européenne) mark in August 2015, allowing commercial sale in European countries.

Bronchoscopic Thermal Vapor Ablation in Clinical Trials

BTVA was first described in 2009 by Snell and colleagues.[30] Eleven patients with severe upper lobe predominant emphysema underwent unilateral BTVA with a mean vapor dose of 4.9 cal/g. At 6 months, TLVR of 16% was observed in MDCT associated with an improvement in health-related quality of life; however, there was no significant change in lung function or exercise tolerance. Based on these data, a high heterogeneity index (HI; tissue-to-air ratio of lower lobe to upper lobe of >1.2) was found to be a significant predictor for good response to BTVA.[31] Eight patients with a high HI experienced greater improvements for FEV_1 and 6-MWT as compared with all 11 patients who underwent BTVA. In the following prospective single-arm trial, 44 patients with predominantly upper lobe emphysema received BTVA with a mean vapor dose of 10 cal/g unilaterally.[32] Six months following BTVA, a TLVR of 48% was noted, leading to a significant improvement of FEV_1 (141 ± 62 mL, $P<.001$), vital capacity (271 ± 72 mL, $P<.001$), and RV (−406 ± 113 mL, $P<.001$). The first RCT is the "Sequential Segmental Treatment of Emphysema With Upper Lobe Predominance Study" known as "Step-Up trial," which was completed in late 2014.[33] In this multicenter prospective trial, 45 patients with upper lobe predominant emphysema underwent bilateral BTVA in a stepwise manner and were compared with 24 patients who received standard medical care. Six months following BTVA, patients of the BTVA group experienced a significant FEV_1 improvement of 13.1% and an SGRQ decrease of 11.1 points.

Complications

The most common adverse event is a local inflammatory reaction (LIR) that can be observed within the first 2 to 4 weeks following BTVA. Patients experience fever, cough, sputum, and dyspnea; an increase of inflammatory markers in the laboratory test; and opacification in the chest radiograph. Therefore, strict monitoring, prophylactic antibiotic therapy, and glucocorticosteroids are crucial to avoid bacterial superinfection and alleviate symptoms. However, the LIR seems to be a prerequisite for the desired TLVR. Patients who develop LIR following BTVA experience a greater clinical outcome than patients without a respiratory adverse event after BTVA.[34] Moreover, the treated lobar volume seems to be a predictor for LIR and thus for outcome. Patients with treated lobar volume greater than 1.700 mL had a high risk of hospitalization due to a respiratory adverse event. However, particularly these patients with a high treated lobar volume developed a TLVR of 73% compared with 40% in patients with treated lobar volume less than 1.700 mL.

Summary

Bronchoscopic thermal vapor ablation presents an effective treatment modality for patients with upper lobe predominant emphysema independent of collateral ventilation. So far, it is the only technique in which no implants are left. The disadvantage, however, is its irreversibility. Thus, a precise patient selection and the search of further predictors for success of BTVA are crucial.

TARGETED LUNG DENERVATION

Targeted Lung Denervation (TLD, Holaira, Minneapolis, MN) is the latest development in the field of endoscopic management of COPD. The aim of TLD is not to reduce hyperinflation, but to minimize bronchoconstriction by ablating parasympathetic innervation of the lungs. Thus, the acetylcholine release that is responsible for smooth muscle contraction is reduced. Therefore, TLD imitates the effect of anticholinergic drugs. TLD is indicated in patients with an FEV_1 of 30% to 60% predicted and positive relative change in FEV_1 of 15% or more following inhalation of ipratropium bromide.

For performing TLD, a dedicated dual-cooled radiofrequency catheter is used. This catheter consists of an electrode that delivers radiofrequency energy, an inflatable balloon at its distal tip, and a coolant that is circulating from an inflow to an outflow conduit. After positioning the catheter in the main bronchi, radiofrequency current with a dose of 15 to 20 Watt passes from the electrode through the bronchi and surrounding tissue. The inner surface of the airway is protected by the coolant and by the inflated balloon that removes heat from the surface of the bronchi wall. To achieve complete circumferential treatment, the electrode must be activated in up to 8 rotational positions. TLD is mainly performed bilaterally in a stepwise manner.

Targeted Lung Denervation in Clinical Trials

So far, there is only 1 prospective single-arm 2-dose pilot trial in which patients with positive response of spirometry to inhaled anticholinergic medication were enrolled.[35] Eleven patients were treated bilaterally by TLD at 20 Watt and 9 patients by TLD at 15 Watt. Efficacy data showed that patients who were treated by the higher power level experienced significant improvements in vital capacity, cycle endurance, and SGRQ. At the lower power level, however, no statistically significant change in any of the clinical measures were observed. Furthermore, it could be demonstrated that the combination of TLD and inhaled anticholinergic drug might result in an increase in FEV_1 over those seen with inhaled muscarinic antagonists alone.

Complications

Slebos and colleagues[35] reported 7 severe adverse events at 1 month following TLD, including COPD exacerbation, anaphylactic drug reaction, coronary artery bypass surgery, chest pain, and gastroparesis. No deaths occurred in that trial. As device-related complications, bronchial perforation, stenosis, and ulceration were detected without the need of intervention. In one case, granulomas were seen that were electively removed by cauterization.

Summary

In conclusion, TLD presents a safe and feasible therapeutic modality for patients with COPD and positive relative change in FEV_1 following administration of muscarinic antagonists. The pilot trial showed encouraging efficacy results, but further investigation of this novel therapy is warranted. Actually, one prospective RCT (Targeted Lung Denervation for Patients With Moderate to Severe COPD), also known as "AIRFLOW-1," is ongoing in Europe.

REFERENCES

1. Gillissen AET. Weißbuch Lunge 2014. Herausforderungen, Zukunftsperspektiven, Forschungsansätze. Zur Lage und Zukunft der Pneumologie in Deutschland. Herne (Westf): FRISCHTEXTE Verlag; 2014.

2. Global strategy for the diagnosis, management and prevention of COPD. Global Initiative for Chronic Obstructive Lung Disease (GOLD); 2015. Available at: http://www.goldcopd.org/.

3. Brantigan OC, Mueller E, Kreis MB. A surgical approach to pulmonary emphysema. Am Rev Respir Dis 1959;80:194–206.

4. Cooper JD, Patterson GA, Sundaresan RS, et al. Results of 150 consecutive bilateral lung volume reduction procedures in patients with severe emphysema. J Thorac Cardiovasc Surg 1996;112:1319–29.

5. Casanova C, Cote C, de Torres JP, et al. Inspiratory-to-total lung capacity radio predicts mortality in patients with chronic obstructive pulmonary disease. Am J Respir Crit Care Med 2005;171:591–7.

6. Fishman A, Martinez F, Naunheim K, et al. A randomized trial comparing lung-volume-reduction surgery with medical therapy for severe emphysema. N Engl J Med 2003;348:2059–73.

7. Sciurba FC, Ernst A, Herth FJF, et al, VENT Study Research Group. A randomized study of endobronchial valves for advanced emphysema. N Engl J Med 2010;363:1233–44.

8. Herth FJ, Noppen M, Valipor A, et al, International VENT Study Group. Efficacy predictors of lung volume reduction with Zephyr valves in a European cohort. Eur Respir J 2012;39:1334–42.

9. Ninane V, Geltner C, Bezzi M, et al. Multicentre European study for the treatment of advanced emphysema with bronchial valves. Respir J 2012;39:1319–25.

10. Eberhardt R, Gompelmann D, Schuhmann M, et al. Complete unilateral vs partial bilateral endoscopic lung volume reduction in patients with bilateral lung emphysema. Chest 2012;142:900–8.

11. Gompelmann D, Eberhardt R, Michaud G, et al. Predicting atelectasis by assessment of collateral ventilation prior to endobronchial lung volume reduction: a feasibility study. Respiration 2010;80:419–25.

12. Herth FJ, Eberhardt R, Gompelmann D, et al. Radiological and clinical outcomes of using Chartis™ to plan endobronchial valve treatment. Eur Respir J 2013;41:302–8.

13. Gompelmann D, Eberhardt R, Slebos DJ, et al. Diagnostic performance comparison of the Chartis system and high-resolution computerized tomography fissure analysis for planning endoscopic lung volume reduction. Respirology 2014;19:524–30.

14. Davey C, Zoumut Z, Jordan S, et al. Bronchoscopic lung volume reduction with endobronchial valves for patients with heterogeneous emphysema and intact interlobar fissures (the BeLieVeR-HIFi study): a randomised controlled trial. Lancet 2015;386(9998):1066–73.

15. Schuhmann M, Raffy P, Yin Y, et al. CT predictors of response to endobronchial valve lung reduction treatment: comparison with Chartis. Am J Respir Crit Care Med 2015;191:767–74.

16. Giesirich W, Kraft M, Reichenberger F, et al. Pneumothorax in treatment of severe emphysema with endobronchial valves. Eur Respir J 2014;9:44.

17. Gompelmann D, Herth FJF, Heussel CP, et al. Pneumothorax nach endoskopischer Ventiltherapie. Pneumologie 2014;68:V454.

18. Bosc C, Jankowski A, Briault A, et al. Long-term outcomes in 35 patients with emphysema after endoscopic lung volume reduction (ELVR) with valves. Eur Respir J 2014;44(Suppl 58):P3734.

19. Gompelmann D, Herth FJF, Slebos DJ, et al. Pneumothorax following endobronchial valve therapy and its impact on clinical outcomes in severe emphysema. Respiration 2014;87:485–91.

20. Herzog D, Poellinger A, Doellinger F, et al. Modifying post-operative medical care after EBV implant may reduce pneumothorax incidence. PLoS One 2015;10:e0128097.

21. Gompelmann D, Eberhardt R, Goldin J, et al. Endoskopische Lungenvolumenreduktion mittels Coil-Implantation bei Patienten mit schwerem heterogenem Lungenemphysem und inkompletten Fissuren: eine retrospektive analyse. DGP 2012 [abstract: 428].

22. Herth FJ, Eberhard R, Gompelmann D, et al. Bronchoscopic lung volume reduction with a dedicated coil: a clinical pilot study. Ther Adv Respir Dis 2010;4:225–31.

23. Slebos DJ, Klooster K, Ernst A, et al. Bronchoscopic lung volume reduction coil treatment of patients with severe heterogeneous emphysema. Chest 2012; 142:574–82.

24. Shah PL, Zoumot Z, Singh S, et al. Endobronchial coils for the treatment of severe emphysema with hyperinflation (RESET): a randomised controlled trial. Lancet Respir Med 2013;1:233–40.

25. Deslee G, Klooster K, Hetzel M, et al. Lung volume reduction coil treatment for patients with severe emphysema: a European multicenter trial. Thorax 2014;69(11):980–6.

26. Klooster K, Ten Hacken NH, Franz I, et al. Lung volume reduction coil treatment in chronic obstructive pulmonary disease patients with homogeneous emphysema: a prospective feasibility trial. Respiration 2014;88:116–25.

27. Hartmann JE, Klooster K, Gortzak K, et al. Long-term follow-up after bronchoscopic lung volume reduction treatment with coils in patients with severe emphysema. Respirology 2015;20: 319–26.

28. Kontogianni K, Gerovasili V, Gompelmann D, et al. Effectiveness and complications of endobronchial coil treatment for lung volume reduction (LVRC) in patients with severe heterogeneous emphysema and bilateral incomplete fissures. Eur Respir J 2014;44(Suppl 58):P1780.

29. Gompelmann D, Heussel CP, Eberhardt R, et al. Efficacy of bronchoscopic thermal vapor ablation and lobar fissure completeness in patients with heterogeneous emphysema. Respiration 2012;83(5): 400–6.

30. Snell GI, Hopkins P, Westall G, et al. A feasibility and safety study of bronchoscopic thermal vapor ablation: a novel emphysema therapy. Ann Thorac Surg 2009;88:1993–8.

31. Herth FJF, Eberhardt R, Ernst A, et al. The efficacy of bronchoscopic thermal vapor ablation in patients with upper lobe emphysema: the impact of heterogeneity of disease. ATS 2010 [abstract: 5167].

32. Snell G, Herth FJ, Hopkins P, et al. Bronchoscopic thermal vapor ablation therapy in the management of heterogeneous emphysema. Eur Respir J 2012; 39(6):1326–33.

33. Herth F, Valipour A, Grah C, et al. Treating the most diseased segments in patients with severe emphysema: 6 months results from the STEP-UP Randomized Controlled Trial (RCT) [abstract 4864]. ERS 2015.

34. Gompelmann D, Eberhardt R, Ernst A, et al. The localized inflammatory response to bronchoscopic thermal vapor ablation. Respiration 2013;86(4): 324–31.

35. Slebos DJ, Klooster K, Koegelenberg CF, et al. Targeted lung denervation for moderate to severe COPD: a pilot study. Thorax 2015;70:411–9.

Advances in Uniportal Video-Assisted Thoracoscopic Surgery
Pushing the Envelope

Diego Gonzalez-Rivas, MD, FECTS[a,b,*], Yang Yang, MD[b],
Calvin NG, MD, FRCS[c]

KEYWORDS

- Uniportal • New technology • Nonintubated lung resection • NOTES • Uniportal sleeve
- 3D camera

KEY POINTS

- The potential benefits of a direct view, anatomic instrumentation, better cosmesis, and potential less postoperative pain have led uniportal video-assisted thoracic surgery to become of increasing interest worldwide.
- The geometric characteristics of the uniportal approach enable expert surgeons to perform complex cases and reconstructive techniques, such as broncho-vascular procedures or carinal resections.
- We can expect more developments of subcostal or embryonic natural orifice translumenal endoscopic surgery access, evolution in anesthesia strategies, and cross-discipline imaging-assisted lesion localization for uniportal procedures.
- The further development of modern 3-dimensional image systems, single-port robotic technology, and wireless cameras in awake or nonintubated patients will probably play an important role in the near future.

 Video content accompanies this article at http://www.thoracic.theclinics.com

INTRODUCTION

Uniportal video-assisted thoracic surgery (VATS) has a history of more than 15 years[1] and, more recently, has become an increasingly popular approach to major pulmonary resections.[2,3] The potential advantages of reduced access trauma, less pain, and better cosmesis, together with patient demand, have seen uniportal VATS spread across the world.[4,5] The early period of uniportal VATS development was focused on procedures such as sympathectomies, pleural deloculations, mediastinal biopsies, bullectomies, and wedge resections for pulmonary nodules.[6–8] The new era of uniportal VATS started in 2010 with the development of the technique for major pulmonary resections.[2] Since then, we have expanded the

Disclosure Statement: The authors have nothing to disclose.
[a] Minimally Invasive Thoracic Surgery Unit (UCTMI), Department of Thoracic Surgery, Coruña University Hospital, Xubias 84, Coruña 15006, Spain; [b] Department of Thoracic Surgery, Shanghai Pulmonary Hospital, Tongji University School of Medicine, 507, Road Zhengmin, Shanghai 200433, China; [c] Division of Cardiothoracic Surgery, The Chinese University of Hong Kong, Prince of Wales Hospital, 30-32 Ngan Shing Street, Shatin, NT, Hong Kong, China
* Corresponding author. Department of Thoracic Surgery, Coruña University Hospital, Xubias 84, Coruña 15006, Spain.
E-mail address: diego.gonzalez.rivas@sergas.es

Thorac Surg Clin 26 (2016) 187–201
http://dx.doi.org/10.1016/j.thorsurg.2015.12.007
1547-4127/16/$ – see front matter © 2016 Elsevier Inc. All rights reserved.

application of this technique to a variety of minimally invasive thoracic surgeries.[9–12] The experience we acquired with the uniportal technique during the past years as well as technological improvements have contributed to the increased adoption of indications for uniportal VATS resections. In only a period of 5 years, experts have been able to apply uniportal VATS technique to encompass more complex procedures such as segmentectomies,[13,14] advanced cases after induction therapies[11] or pneumonectomies,[15,16] and even to challenging procedures including bronchial sleeve,[17–19] vascular reconstructions,[12,20] carinal resections,[12] or double sleeves.[12,21,22] The large number of surgical videos posted on the Internet, live surgery events, and experimental courses have also contributed to the rapid expansion of uniportal VATS during the past years. Training and adoption of the technique in more thoracic departments and outcome reports for long-term survival and oncological benefits are necessary to reinforce the worldwide adoption of this approach. The 5-year overall survival and disease-free survival in our series of patients with stage IA of non–small-cell lung cancer (NSCLC) was 90% and 75%, respectively.[23]

As with any recent approach for lung cancer treatment, safety and efficacy are paramount. Studies so far have shown the uniportal VATS approach to be at least as safe and effective as conventional VATS.[24] Postoperative pain has been shown to be less following uniportal VATS lung resection when compared with multiportal VATS,[9] and current data show at least equivalent disease-free survival at intermediate follow-up for patients with early-stage NSCLC who received uniportal VATS surgery.[25] We believe it is important to minimize the surgical aggressiveness, especially in patients with advanced-stage lung cancer in whom the immune system is weakened by the disease or by induction treatments. The minimally invasive surgery represents the least aggressive form to operate lung cancer and the uniportal technique is the final evolution in these minimally invasive surgical techniques.[26]

The main advances of uniportal VATS during the past years are related to improvements in surgical technique and implementation of new technology (better staplers and energy devices, 3-dimensional [3D] and ultra–high-definition view). The experience gained during the past years has allowed refinement of the technique to develop tricks to easily manage the upper lobe vein and bronchus (both being the most difficult structures to divide), to use energy devices for hilar dissection, and to control most of the intraoperative bleeding. The uniportal approach also facilitates the

performance of radical lymphadenectomies and reconstructive complex tracheo-bronchial and vascular procedures. Furthermore, the use of a single incision can be combined with nonintubated techniques as well used for major pulmonary resections through a subxiphoid incision.

IMPROVEMENTS IN SURGICAL TECHNIQUE: DEVELOPMENT OF USEFUL TRICKS
Upper Lobe Vein Division

The most difficult structure to divide through a single-incision approach is the upper lobe vein. It is also the most frequent reason for conversion to a multiport approach during the learning curve. The uniportal view facilitates the dissection and division of the upper arterial trunk, usually hidden by the superior vein when we use a conventional thoracoscopic approach. Once the arterial branch is divided, it is important to dissect the vein as distal as possible to optimize passage of the stapler. We recommend encircling of the vein by using a vessel loop for upper lobectomies. Pulling the vein enlarges the space and clears the vision for stapler insertion.

A useful trick to facilitate the passage of the stapler is to insert the curved tip suction device behind the vein. By doing this maneuver, the suction device serves as a guide and the artery is protected when the stapler is inserted (**Fig. 1**, Video 1).

Yang and colleagues[27] used a Foley catheter to guide the endostapler to the right position and Guo and colleagues[28] described a method of intrathoracic vertical overhanging approach to make the placement of the endostapler easier during single-port VATS lobectomy.

The use of the curved-tip stapler technology (Covidien, Mansfield, MA) clearly facilitates the passage around the artery and superior pulmonary vein through a single incision. The new vascular powered staplers, more narrow (7 mm) and with a curved tip (Ethicon Endo-Surgery Inc, Cincinnati, OH) or the 80° angulated 5-mm curved-tip staplers (microCutter Xchange 30; Cardica, Inc., Redwood City, CA, USA) are an excellent option for the uniportal approach and especially useful for the management of the upper vein.

If, despite using these tricks, there are still difficulties in dividing the vein, then the use of a conventional TA stapler (2 cartridges) is an easy alternative and a valid option, especially useful during the learning curve.[29] Another option is to approach the vein with the angulation of the tip of the stapler oriented to the fissure (**Fig. 2**). If the fissure is complete, the passage is easier with this orientation. In case of incomplete fissure,

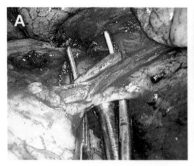 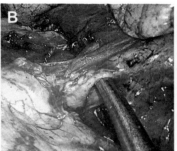 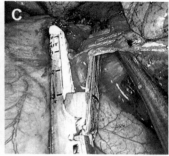

Fig. 1. Surgical trick to facilitate the stapler insertion to the left upper lobe vein: (*A*) vein dissection, (*B*) curved tip suction device as a path to protect the insertion of the stapler to divide the vein (*C*).

we must first open the fissure from the hilum to create a tunnel between the upper and lower vein with identification of the bronchus and artery. The anvil of the stapler is placed over the artery, dividing the anterior portion of the fissure and allowing for the mobilization of the lobe (to allow the stapling of the vein from the opposite angle).

Left Upper Lobe Bronchus

The dissection and division of the left upper lobe bronchus also can be difficult. It can be done in 3 ways when experience is acquired with the technique.

The first option is to open the fissure from the hilum, as previously described, to expose and divide the lingular artery, and then insert an endostapler for the bronchus. The second option is to use a TA stapler (2 cartridges), and the third option is by cutting the bronchus with scissors and suturing at the end.

Regardless of this, if after 10 minutes of unsuccessfully trying to insert the staplers for the upper lobe vein or bronchus, it is recommended to add another incision just to insert the stapler. Once the vein or bronchus is divided, surgeons can continue the operation safely with the uniportal approach. Forcing the insertion of the stapler can cause injury to the artery, resulting in major bleeding with catastrophic consequences. Once experience is gained with the uniportal approach, the second incision may not be necessary.

Camera and Instrumentation Management

The placement of the incision is crucial during the uniportal approach and usually is located more anterior, at the fifth intercostal space (fourth intercostal space is more suitable for Right upper lobes).[6] The surgeon and the assistant usually stand on the anterior side of the patient and their position can be exchanged during the procedure depending on whether the upper or lower lobe is to be resected, so as to facilitate instrumentation and view.[24]

Placing the camera in the posterior part of the incision is one of the most important aspects to obtain an anatomic view and a proper instrumentation, working with the instruments below (same concept as open surgery). Stabilizing the camera may be challenging, because the trocar is not used during uniportal VATS. The use of a suture around the camera to pull the camera backward is helpful to maintain the position of the camera posteriorly to the patient. It is also convenient to use a lateral suture to keep the lung-retracting grasper steady to expose the hilum (**Fig. 3**A).

To avoid inflation of the lung when we use suction, 2 lateral sutures can be placed pulling the soft tissue to keep the incision open. Occasionally it is useful to place a gauze between the camera and the posterior part of incision to prevent blood from dripping onto the tip of the thoracoscope (**Fig. 3**B).

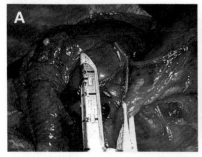 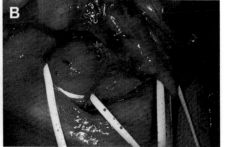

Fig. 2. Surgical image showing unusual stapler angulation for a right upper lobe vein (*A*), and left upper lobe vein (*B*).

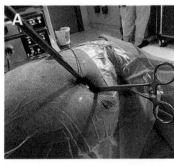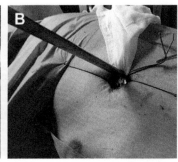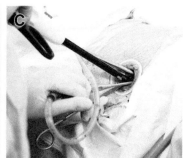

Fig. 3. Photo showing the surgical incision. (*A*) A suture is placed to keep the camera in the posterior part of the incision. (*B*) Two lateral sutures are placed to retract the soft tissue from the incision. (*C*) Surgical instrumentation through a wound protector.

A wound protector is routinely not used in our practice because the plastic ring inside may diminish instrument manipulation, especially when adhesions are present. They may be used though, for sleeve resections or very obese patients as in these cases optimal instrumentation may be challenging (**Fig. 3**C). However, it is recommended to use the wound protector during the learning curve. Once experience is gained, the use of the wound protector may be minimized.

Energy Devices for Vascular Dissection and Division

The most frequent use of ultrasonic energy devices during VATS procedures is for the release of lung adhesions or to facilitate lymph node dissection. Although ultrasound energy devices may cause thermal injuries near vascular structures, they can be used safely and efficiently in expert hands. These devices offer cutting, coagulation, dissecting, and grasping all in one. The versatility and safety profiles make ultrasonic energy a compelling technology to consider for uniportal VATS lobectomy (Video 2). It is important to be extremely cautious to avoid thermal injuries during vascular dissection.[30]

The metal or polymer clips are a safe and a cheap option to divide small pulmonary vessels (**Fig. 4**). The new specifically designed 45° applier for uniportal VATS (Click aV; Grena, Brentford, UK) is helpful during uniportal surgery. The use of 2 clips for the proximal end of small branches and the use of energy devices or ligation to cut the distal end of the vessel is recommended (see **Fig. 4**). There are 2 reasons for doing this: to avoid the accidental displacement of the distal clips while manipulating the lobe and to prevent the clip from getting in the middle of the stapler line when dividing the fissure. Sealing the vessel at a distal end adds more safety to prevent the proximal stump from bleeding in case of a displaced clip.[31] The use of a suture to tie the segmental vessels is also a safe, cheap, and valid option when using a thoracoscopic knot pusher (Video 3).

Lymph Node Dissection

The thoracoscope inserted through the single incision provides the operator with an excellent ergonomic view to reach the retro-cava space or even the left side of the upper mediastinum during an extended right-side upper mediastinal lymph node dissection. The way to perform a complete

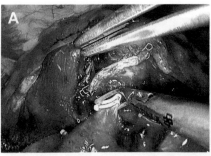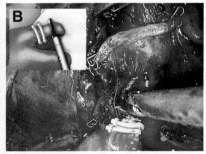

Fig. 4. Surgical image showing (*A*) the use of polymer clips for proximal division of segmental artery during left upper lobectomy and (*B*) the use of energy devices for distal division of the vessel.

lymph node dissection is similar to the multiport technique. However, some conditions and special techniques are required to achieve a radical lymphadenectomy, including the use of modified instruments, such as longer and curved tip suckers and double-joint thoracoscopic instruments to avoid instrument clashing. High-definition cameras improve the view to detect small and deep lymph nodes and energy devices facilitate a more radical, safe, and less bloody lymph node dissection (Video 4).

The most difficult areas, such as the left paratracheal and left subcarinal space, can be totally dissected with an improved view in the uniportal technique (see Video 4). The use of a sponge stick to retract the lung enlarges the subcarinal space. Bimanual instrumentation using a long curved tip suction on the left hand and energy devices on the right hand clearly facilitate the procedure and diminish the incidence of bleeding during dissection. The suction device is helpful for blunt dissection and blood removal. For hilar and N1 station lymphadenectomy, it is important to move and rotate the operating table posteriorly so as to place the lung in the back position. For right or left paratracheal dissection, the anti-Trendelenburg position is helpful because it naturally makes the lung "fall down." For subcarinal dissection, the Trendelenburg position and the anterior table rotation facilitate the exposure. Preliminary division of the pulmonary ligament gives us a better access to the subcarinal space as well.[32]

Bleeding Control

The correct assessment of any bleeding is paramount during uniportal thoracoscopic major procedures.[31,33] If bleeding occurs, a sponge stick should be readily available to apply pressure immediately to control the hemorrhage. After initial compression with a sponge stick, the use of the suction device is helpful to compress the bleeding site and to keep the bleeding site clear of blood. A curved tip suction device does not interfere with the suturing maneuver or the thoracoscopic view through a single-port approach.

It is not recommended to apply a thoracoscopic clamp directly to the injury because the defect can be enlarged. If the bleeding does not stop after initial compression, it can be useful to use an atraumatic instrument, such as a ring forceps or vascular clamp, to grasp the artery and stop the bleeding as a first step, and then perform a thoracoscopic repair by means of suture. In the event of a significant defect, it is ideal to isolate the main pulmonary artery with the use of a clamp or a vessel loop to suppress the afferent vascular flow (Video 5). This allows us to better assess the defect and apply the suture with more precision and safety. To repair the defect through a uniportal approach, bimanual instrumentation is crucial, keeping the camera at the posterior position and the instruments at the anterior position. This enables a very direct vision of the bleeding site, and similar maneuvers, as in open surgery, can be reproduced. The preferred method to suture the pulmonary artery is to use the thoracoscopic curved suction in the left hand and the needle holder in the right hand (**Fig. 5**). In the case of frail injured vessels or a significant laceration on the base of the main pulmonary artery, it is recommended to reinforce the suture with Teflon patches.[31]

Even though most of vascular injuries can be controlled by VATS when in expert hands, there are some situations that can require conversion to a thoracotomy, such as major uncontrollable bleeding. Panic can result in an initial small injury turning into a more significant defect after failed attempts to control the bleeding through the use of clamps or unsuccessful sutures.

The conversion to open surgery should never be considered as a failure of VATS, but rather as a form of guaranteeing the safety of the patient. It is essential to know at which moment the surgery should be converted and this will depend on the experience of each surgeon. The advantage of the uniportal approach is the swiftness to which it can be converted to an open thoracotomy, by enlarging the incision, which is usually placed at the fifth intercostal space.

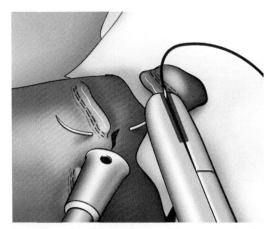

Fig. 5. Drawing showing bimanual instrumentation for bleeding control and suturing of the pulmonary artery.

NONINTUBATED MAJOR PULMONARY RESECTIONS: REDUCING TRAUMA TO THE PATIENT

The main advantage of nonintubated surgery is to avoid the perioperative morbidity derived from the deleterious effect of general anesthesia and 1-lung ventilation, in addition to the beneficial effects of spontaneous ventilation in a nonintubated patient.[34–36]

Inclusion criteria for a nonintubated uniportal procedure includes all selected patients for whom the avoidance of morbidity of conventional thoracotomy and the risk of intubated general anesthesia could be reduced.[37]

The choice of a single incision technique in an awake or nonintubated patient could minimize the invasiveness of the procedure[38] (Fig. 6). This combination could be appropriate in high-risk patients for general intubated anesthesia, such as elderly patients or those with poor pulmonary function.[39] It is advisable to perform a careful selection of the patients, especially during the learning curve. The contraindications for awake major resections are patients with an expected difficult airway management, obesity (body mass index >30), dense and extensive pleural adhesions, hemodynamically unstable patients, ASA >II, and large tumors (>6 cm).[40]

Thanks to the avoidance of intubation, mechanical ventilation, and muscle relaxants, the anesthetic side effects are minimal, allowing most of the patients to be included in a fast protocol avoiding the stay in an intensive care unit. Moreover, the perioperative surgical stress response could be attenuated in nonintubated patients undergoing uniportal VATS as a result of the reduced postoperative stress hormones and proinflammatory mediators related to mechanical ventilation. Oxygen (6–9 L/min) is supplied via nasal cannulae or facial mask. The pharmacologic management is based on a target-controlled infusion of remifentanil and propofol, with a premedication of midazolam (0.15–0.25 mg/kg) and atropine (0.01 mg/kg) 15 minutes before anesthesia, adjusting the real-time rate of infusion with the aggressiveness of each period during the surgery. The use of an intraoperative vagus blockade suppresses coughing that could be troublesome when performing lung traction and hilar manipulation during dissection.

When performing a uniportal approach in a nonintubated patient, it is necessary to perform a paravertebral blockade or an intercostal infiltration under thoracoscopic view[41] (Video 6). The importance of avoiding epidural thoracic blockade (avoiding opioids) will result in faster recovery and return to daily activities.

The nonintubated VATS major pulmonary resections must be performed only in collaboration with experienced anesthesiologists and uniportal thoracoscopic surgeons (preferably skilled and experienced with complex or advanced cases as well as bleeding control through VATS). However, intraoperative conversion to general anesthesia is sometimes necessary. The anesthesiologist must be skilled in bronchoscopic intubation, placing a double-lumen tube or an endobronchial blocker in a lateral decubitus position.[40]

RECONSTRUCTIVE TECHNIQUES: PUSHING THE LIMITS

One of the most recent advances in the uniportal VATS approach is the possibility of performing reconstructive broncho-vascular techniques to avoid pneumonectomies.[12,17–22] Complex lung resections, including thoracoscopic double sleeve, bronchial-sparing lung resections, and tracheal or carinal reconstructions have been reported by experts in the field.[12]

Performing the incision at the fourth or fifth intercostal space, more anteriorly (anterior axillary line), facilitates the positioning of the needle holder

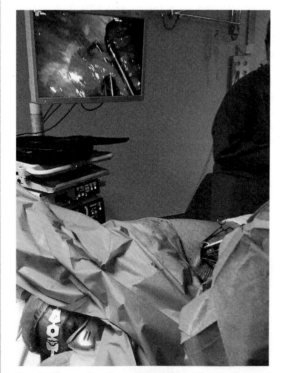

Fig. 6. Photo showing surgical instrumentation and anesthetic management (bispectral index and facial mask) during a nonintubated uniportal VATS left lower lobectomy.

parallel to the hilum, making suturing similar to an open anterior thoracotomy. When performing bronchial suturing using uniportal VATS, it is important to maintain the camera on the posterior of the patient, operating with both hands below the camera (bimanual instrumentation). This is the same principle as when performing an anterior thoracotomy in open surgery: direct view with the surgeon's eyes above his or her hands.[12] The geometric explanation of the approach[42] and the ergonomics[43] are important factors to facilitate the sleeve reconstructions through a uniportal approach. As a result, in expert hands, the anastomosis can be accomplished from a straight perspective. Using a wound protector is helpful when dealing with obese patients because fatty tissue could interfere with the suture threads. The positioning of the operating table helps to expose the lung and so it is easier to perform the anastomosis (the 45° rotation of the table toward the surgeon positions the lung anteriorly and makes the posterior bronchial suturing easier, especially the membranous portion).

The sleeve anastomosis can be performed with interrupted or continuous suture. Placing interrupted sutures by VATS can be more complex and time-consuming. Our preferred method is to use a continuous absorbable suture (Polydioxanone, PDS 3/0; Ethicon, Johnson & Johnson, New Brunswick, NJ, USA), which makes the thread movement easier, as well as the tying. Our personal technique for uniportal thoracoscopic suture is for the surgeon to tie the knot outside of the chest, holding both ends of the thread with the left hand's index and pinkie fingers and pushing down the knots with a thoracoscopic knot pusher.[12,44] The anastomosis also can be performed by using a novel absorbable barbed suture, the V-Loc wound closure device (Covidien), which avoids knot-tying and keeps strength and security[45] and makes the running suture easy. This suture is useful when dealing with a complex anastomosis, deeply located (Video 7).

For double sleeve procedures, the use of a thoracoscopic clamp for the main pulmonary artery and a bulldog clamp for the distal end of the vessel is the most appropriate choice (**Fig. 7**A) The arterial clamp is placed in the anterior portion of the incision and the camera always at the posterior aspect of the patient. This makes the bronchial and arterial anastomoses more comfortable.[12,21,22]

VATS lung-sparing bronchial sleeve resection and reconstructions are technically more challenging than a standard VATS sleeve lobectomy (**Fig. 7**B). The bronchial anastomosis after a VATS sleeve lobectomy is less complex to perform because there is more space to expose the 2 bronchial ends for suturing once the lobe has been removed.[12,46]

Tumors involving the trachea or carina pose many challenges during thoracoscopic surgery, as it requires a total coordination with the anesthesiologist.[47] A precise airway management and reconstruction and a preoperative plan in case of emergency is required. To perform this procedure through uniportal VATS[44] there are 2 options to maintain lung ventilation: the use of an intra–surgical field tracheal tube[48] or through a high-frequency jet ventilation[49] (**Fig. 8**) (see Video 7). The latter can be introduced through the endotracheal tube and thanks to the small diameter of the catheter for ventilation, it does not interfere with the anastomosis of the membranous portion (**Fig. 7**D). This way we do not need intrafield intubation. In the event of needing surgical field intubation, a sterile circuit is passed onto the field and prepared to directly ventilate a single lung (through the same incision or adding a second small port)[12] (**Fig. 7**C).

SUBXIPHOID APPROACH: A NOVEL CONCEPT

Recent innovations in the single-incision approach include the use of the subxiphoid technique for major resections (**Fig. 9**).[50] Avoiding the incision through the intercostal space could be another potential advantage to reduce postoperative pain, but further studies will be required to demonstrate that this approach is less painful. This approach has been used during the past years for different thoracic procedures, such as pericardial window, thymectomy, or pulmonary metastasectomy, and recently was introduced for bilateral resections. Liu[51] reported in 2013 the first case of thoracoscopic lobectomy with mediastinal lymph node sampling through a single subxiphoid incision for patients with lung cancer.

This approach has several limitations, such as the handling of major bleeding. When an emergent conversion to open surgery is necessary, an extension of the subxiphoid incision is unlikely to be useful and an additional thoracotomy should be performed.

Moreover, a complete lymphadenectomy is difficult to achieve via the subxiphoid approach and there is limited access to posterior anatomy. From the subxiphoid to the hilum, it is in an oblique and longer distance, so the instrument-fighting problem during uniportal surgery will be even more challenging than those with a transthoracic approach. The instrumentation over the beating heart is also bothering, especially during left side procedures. Further studies are needed to document the applicability and compare clinical outcomes of the uniportal subxiphoid versus the

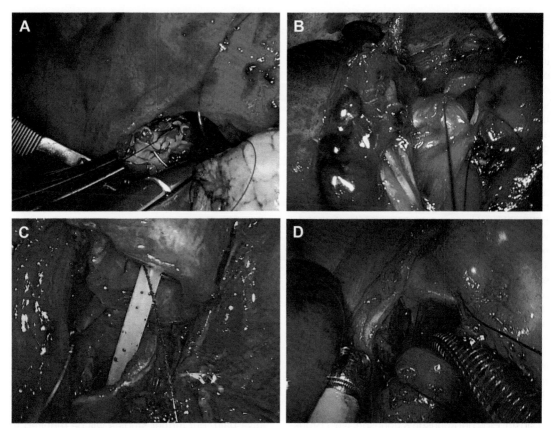

Fig. 7. Surgical image showing complex uniportal procedures. (*A*) Vascular anastomosis during a double-sleeve resection. (*B*) Bronchial sleeve anastomosis after carcinoid tumor resection located in the bronchus intermedius. (*C*) Anastomosis of the trachea to the left main bronchus after right carinal pneumonectomy (under high-frequency ventilation jet). (*D*) Distal tracheal resection and reconstruction (intrafield intubation to ventilate the left main bronchus).

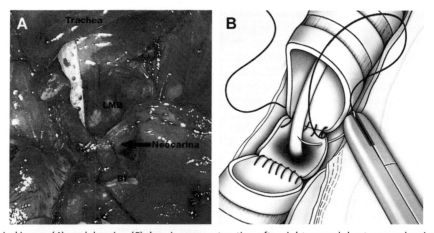

Fig. 8. Surgical image (*A*), and drawing (*B*) showing reconstruction after right upper lobectomy and carinal resection (under high-frequency jet ventilation of the left lung): lateral wall of the left main bronchus is anastomosed to the lateral wall of trachea. A neocarina is then created with left main bronchus and bronchus intermedius. The anastomosis is completed by anterior and posterior running sutures. BI, bronchus intermedius; LMB, left main bronchus.

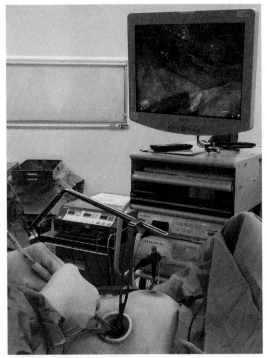

Fig. 9. Subxiphoid approach for a VATS right middle lobectomy.

transthoracic approach, so as to show benefits from this technique.

VISUALIZING SURGERY

Perhaps the single most important technological advancement that allowed the development of minimally invasive thoracic surgery was the rod lens thoracoscope. Not only did it allow the surgeon to see the operating field by "going inside" the thoracic cavity, but in addition provided image clarity and magnification, as well as alternate viewing angles that even open surgery cannot match. In uniportal VATS, all the instruments are crowded into a single incision, resulting in instrument fencing. Furthermore, there is no longer the option of changing instrument positions by placing the thoracoscope in another port to gain better visualization. Improved viewing angles during uniportal VATS can be achieved by using a 30° lens, a thinner 5-mm scope, and changing the position of the thoracoscope in relation to the other instruments within the single incision.[52] However, vision toward the posterior part of the operating field can remain challenging. The new generation of thoracoscopes provides variable angle technology that allow zero to 120° range of vision. The wide viewing angle gives unparalleled vision to the whole pleural cavity, and in addition avoids

torqueing of the scope at the incision site.[53] Furthermore, the tip of the thoracoscope can be positioned away from the operating site, minimizing fencing with other endoscopic instruments and freeing up more instrument operating space.[52] The 2 most commonly used designs for the wide variable angle thoracoscopes include a rigid rod with an end rotating prism versus an end deflectable flexible bronchoscopy tip. In general, the former has a wider shaft and produces a less bright image, whereas the latter has a more fragile tip design and the deflected tip may interfere with the operating instruments.[53] As alternate access approaches to uniportal VATS, such as subxiphoid or even axillary incision, continue to be explored to minimize intercostal nerve injury and further improve cosmesis, the wide varying angle lens thoracoscopes may play an even more important role in facilitating the surgery.[54]

Another recent development is 3-dimensional (3D) imaging of intrathoracic structures using a double lens binocular system. Interestingly, such 3D technology has been used in the cinema for almost 3 decades, making its major debut in Hollywood movies. As the technology matured, the earlier problems of excessively heavy 3D glasses and camera heads, dimmer images compared with 2D systems, sterilization compatibility, and prohibitively high costs are no longer issues. However, even with current technology, independent scope rotation associated with changes in visual horizon can distort the 3D images, resulting in loss of definition. Three-dimensional technology has the potential advantages of improving visualization by restoring natural 3D vision and depth perception, and thereby facilitating faster and more accurate grasping, suturing, and dissection during surgery. Furthermore, it may help to accelerate the learning curve for surgical tasks. The use of high-definition 3D imaging has been applied to wide varying degree thoracoscopes[55] (**Fig. 10**).

In terms of having the ideal thoracoscope and future developments, over the years several concepts have emerged. The idea of integrating the thoracoscope into surgical instruments during uniportal VATS would be a solution to reduce instrument fencing and may potentially lead to a smaller incision. Perhaps the first realization of this approach was in 2002 when Lardinois and Ris[56] published their experience of using the modified pediatric cystoresectoscope for uniportal sympathectomy. Subsequently, more modern variations of the same design have been reported, including the use of an endoscopic vein harvesting device to perform uniportal VATS.[57,58] In recent years, the development of uniportal robotic

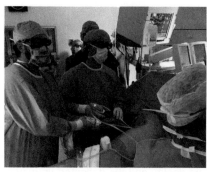
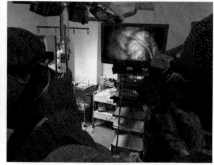

Fig. 10. Uniportal VATS lobectomy with 3D thoracoscope.

technology and endoscopes for natural orifice transumbilical endoscopic surgery (NOTES) also follows the same philosophy of thoracoscopic integration with surgical instruments, and these will be discussed later in this article.

Another interesting future development is the wireless (or cableless) thoracoscope. The concept was initially presented in the "air-scope" design with a self-LED illumination, and a wireless antenna to remotely transmit signal and images.[59] Such a design will allow the clutter associated with light and transmission cables to be removed, and at the same time provide unrestrained movement of the thoracoscope. Subsequently, others have explored the possibility of a small clip-on wireless "capsule" remote video camera placed on a surgical instrument, for example, at the end of an endoscopic energy dissecting device.[60] However, this approach was quickly dismissed due to the movement artifact presented to the camera by the surgical instrument during the surgical procedure. The evolution of this design took the remote video camera away from being attached to the surgical instruments but instead being attached to the chest wall. Ironically, the ribs and rigid thoracic cage presented thoracic surgeons with challenges in terms of access

and specimen retrieval, among others,[61] and yet it can provide a very stable platform to "mount" the remote video camera. The magnetic anchoring guidance system (MAGS) concept uses magnets placed on the outer surface of the chest wall to hold and control a small remote camera within the chest cavity to visualize surgery.[60] The advantages include a large viewing angle, as the camera can potentially be magnetically attached to most areas of the chest wall, and also the wireless remote design will not occupy the incision space nor cause instrument fencing. The latest design of the MAGS camera (**Fig. 11**) is more compact and ergonomic to insert and glide over the inner chest wall. Furthermore, because there are no wires to clutter the operating space, potentially multiple cameras can be inserted into the chest cavity to provide panoramic views of the operating field (**Fig. 12**). Other imaging technologies in development that can enhance minimally invasive thoracic surgery, although not exclusively for uniportal, include preoperative 3D HRCT (3 dimensional high resolution computed tomography) reconstruction with 3D thoracoscopic image overlay and fluorescence luminescence with thoracoscopic image overlay.[62] These imaging modalities can improve the

Fig. 11. MAGS camera with wireless and remote transmission and steerable control.

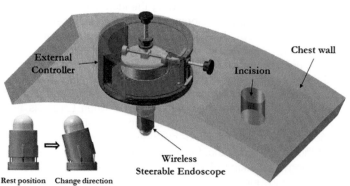

US Patent pending

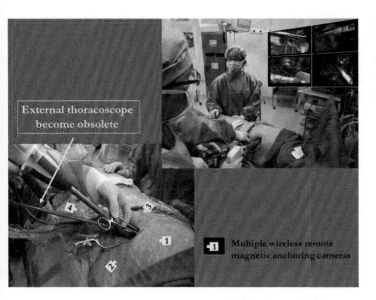

Fig. 12. Illustrated photo of multiple remote wireless cameras, such as the MAGS camera, positioned inside the thoracic cavity providing simultaneously different views of the operating field. The thoracoscope cables may become obsolete (*red arrows*).

identification of lung lesions and hilar structures (segmental airways and vessels), as well as potentially provide important information on adequacy of resection margins resulting in better and safer surgery. The way surgeons look at surgical pathology within the chest will change significantly in the coming decade.

UNIPORTAL VATS: NOT AS WE KNOW IT

As uniportal VATS surgery calls for flexible thinking and new direction of approach to minimally invasive thoracic surgery, it has contributed to fueling the interest in development of other forms of single access instrument platforms, such as embryonic NOTES (e-NOTES) and single-incision robotic surgery, which may well have significant roles in the thoracic surgery of the future.[54,60,63]

The use of NOTES as a platform to access the chest for thoracic procedures would probably remain in the realms of the most adventurous thoracic surgeons for some time to come. Nevertheless, NOTES via the trans-tracheal route has been performed in the animal swine model.[64] Perhaps a more acceptable approach is e-NOTES, which uses the "embryonic natural orifice," the umbilicus, to execute simple uniportal thoracic procedures. In 2013, Zhu and colleagues[65] reported their initial experience of e-NOTES for thoracic sympathectomy in patients suffering from palmar hyperhidrosis. The transumbilical e-NOTES approach used a 5-mm ultrathin flexible gastroscope, using a needle knife to create an opening in the diaphragm to reach the pleural space. Various standard

endoscopic tools, including electrocautery forceps, could be deployed to perform the thoracic sympathectomy. In their latest experience of 35 patients who received the e-NOTES thoracic sympathectomy, the success rate was 97% at 1 year, with no operative or delayed complications. The patients reported less pain and higher satisfaction with the aesthetic results when compared with conventional needlescopic VATS sympathectomy.[66] Since the success of e-NOTES sympathectomy, other procedures, including e-NOTES pericardial window and wedge lung resection, have been reported[67]; however, a more sophisticated endoscopic platform is required for future development of more complex thoracic procedures. Some of the better known developments in these advance flexible endoscopic platforms are EndoSamurai (Olympus, Tokyo, Japan), Anubiscope (Karl Storz, Tuttlingen, Germany), TransPort (USGI Medical, San Clemente, CA), Cobra (USGI Medical), and Direct Drive Endoscopic System (Boston Scientific, Marlborough, Massachusetts, USA). These platforms possess a steerable endoscopic component, some of which have an endoscope conformation fixation feature. Furthermore, the multiple large channels allow utilization of NOTES tools that can be individually controlled to gain instrument triangulation.[60,68] The needle cautery, endoscopic graspers, cautery, and clips within the directable instrument arms provide superb manual dexterity, ergonomics, and control for the operator and hence allow more complex procedures to be performed. In addition, the operator has the ability to exert traction and countertraction on tissues through a single endoscopic port. The use of these advance NOTES/e-NOTES platforms for more complex thoracic procedures will require further refinement and future development.

When discussing NOTES for the chest, it is often easy to forget that pulmonary lesions can be reached via navigating the airways. Although the consequences of breeching a major airway such as trachea or main bronchus is severe, "operating" through the minor airways can be the ideal access for NOTES in treating lung pathologies. In recent years, electromagnetic navigational bronchoscopy (ENB) has slowly become accepted as a tool for the biopsy of small peripheral lung lesions. Using real-time electromagnetic guidance based on preoperative 3D reconstructed computed tomography imaging, the system guides the operator through the small distal airways by a navigational catheter directly to the pulmonary lesion for diagnostic biopsy. Lately, the indications for ENB has expanded to dye marking to aid pulmonary nodule localization during minimally invasive VATS surgery, and metallic fiducial implantation primarily for specialized radiotherapy techniques, such as cyberknife therapy. As technology continues to rapidly evolve, therapeutic tools such as radiofrequency or microwave ablation probes, photodynamic therapy catheters, or even micro-instrumentation endoscopic arms may be available through the ENB that allow perhaps small lesions or nonsurgical candidates to be treated through this ultimate NOTES platform. As previously mentioned, the use of real-time imaging in the hybrid operating theater setting will likely play a key role in guiding and confirming ENB-directed therapy.

The current DaVinci robotic system is a major advance in thoracic surgery by providing excellent 3D visual feedback coupled with robotic arm dexterity and precision; however, most systems require operating through multiple ports.[60] Despite recent developments in robotic single-incision laparoscopic surgery (SILS) by operating through special SILS ports with computer-compensated movements for instrument crossover, the process is difficult and is not popular. Using the present robotic platform, robotic SILS probably represents the limit for the current system design in terms of minimizing surgical access trauma. To minimize access trauma via a single-incision approach and to be able to perform complex skills, the whole functional aspects of the robot, namely the robot's "shoulders," "arms," and "head and eyes" need to be folded and inserted within the operating cavity. The latest DaVinci single-port robotic system uses a 2.5-cm diameter insertable platform that opens up within the operating cavity into a steerable 3D

camera and 3 effector arms for tissue handling and suturing. Other promising system designs based on similar philosophy include the Insertable Robotic Effector Platform (IREP) developed by Columbia University,[69] and the KidsArm System developed by the Center for Image-Guided Innovation and Therapeutic Intervention at the Hospital for Sick Children in Toronto. These designs also hold great promise as ultrathin subcentimeter insertable platforms are developed with noncompromising 3D vision and dexterous surgical arms that allow retraction and suturing with amazing positional accuracy of 0.25 mm or less, potentially allowing even microsurgical procedures to be performed. These systems will no doubt be the next generation of surgical robots that will totally transform and redefine minimally invasive single-incision thoracic surgery.

SUMMARY

The uniportal approach has created new opportunities for collaboration with the industry to push the boundaries on minimally invasive surgery. During the past years a rapid progress in instrument design and technology has taken place. We expect further developments, such as narrower and more angulated endostaplers, sealing devices for vessels, and fissure and refined thoracoscopic instruments. The improvements in 3D systems, wireless cameras, and robotic surgery, may allow the uniportal approach to become more widely available for thoracic surgeons.

SUPPLEMENTARY DATA

Supplementary data related to this article can be found at http://dx.doi.org/10.1016/j.thorsurg.2015.12.007.

REFERENCES

1. Lin TS, Kuo SJ, Chou MC. Uniportal endoscopic thoracic sympathectomy for treatment of palmar and axillary hyperhidrosis: analysis of 2000 cases. Neurosurgery 2002;51:84–7.
2. Gonzalez D, Paradela M, Garcia J, et al. Single-port video-assisted thoracoscopic lobectomy. Interact Cardiovasc Thorac Surg 2011;12:514–5.
3. Gonzalez-Rivas D, Fernandez R, de la Torre M, et al. Thoracoscopic lobectomy through a single incision. Multimed Man Cardiothorac Surg 2012;2012: mms007.
4. Rocco G. One-port (uniportal) video-assisted thoracic surgical resections: a clear advance. J Thorac Cardiovasc Surg 2012;144(3):S27–31.
5. Gonzalez-Rivas D, Fieira E, Delgado M, et al. Evolving from conventional video-assisted

thoracoscopic lobectomy to uniportal: the story behind the evolution. J Thorac Dis 2014;6(S6):S599–603.

6. Rocco G, Martin-Ucar A, Passera E. Uniportal VATS wedge pulmonary resections. Ann Thorac Surg 2004;77:726.

7. Rocco G, Brunelli A, Jutley R, et al. Uniportal VATS for mediastinal nodal diagnosis and staging. Interact Cardiovasc Thorac Surg 2006;5:430–2.

8. Jutley RS, Khalil MW, Rocco G. Uniportal vs standard three-port VATS technique for spontaneous pneumothorax: comparison of post-operative pain and residual paraesthesia. Eur J Cardiothorac Surg 2005;28:43–6.

9. Gonzalez-Rivas D, Paradela M, Fernandez R, et al. Uniportal video-assisted thoracoscopic lobectomy: two years of experience. Ann Thorac Surg 2013;95:426–32.

10. Gonzalez-Rivas D, Fieira E, Delgado M, et al. Is uniportal thoracoscopic surgery a feasible approach for advanced stages of non-small cell lung cancer? J Thorac Dis 2014;6(6):641–8.

11. Gonzalez-Rivas D, Fieira E, Delgado M, et al. Uniportal video-assisted thoracoscopic sleeve lobectomy and other complex resections. J Thorac Dis 2014;6(S6):674–81.

12. Gonzalez-Rivas D, Yang Y, Stupnik T, et al. Uniportal video-assisted thoracoscopic bronchovascular, tracheal and carinal resections. Eur J Cardiothorac Surg 2016;49:i6–16.

13. Gonzalez-Rivas D, Fieira E, Mendez L, et al. Single port video-assisted thoracoscopic segmentectomy and right upper lobectomy. Eur J Cardiothorac Surg 2012;42(6):e169–71.

14. Gonzalez-Rivas D. Single incision video-assisted thoracoscopic anatomic segmentectomy. Ann Cardiothorac Surg 2014;3(2):204–7.

15. Gonzalez-Rivas D, De la Torre M, Fernandez R, et al. Single-incision video-assisted thoracoscopic right pneumonectomy. Surg Endosc 2012;26(7):2078–9.

16. Gonzalez-Rivas D, Delgado M, Fieira E, et al. Uniportal video-assisted thoracoscopic pneumonectomy. J Thorac Dis 2013;5(Suppl 3):S246–52.

17. Gonzalez-Rivas D, Fernandez R, Fieira E, et al. Uniportal video-assisted thoracoscopic bronchial sleeve lobectomy: first report. J Thorac Cardiovasc Surg 2013;145(6):1676–7.

18. Gonzalez-Rivas D, Delgado M, Fieira E, et al. Left lower sleeve lobectomy by uniportal video-assisted thoracoscopic approach. Interact Cardiovasc Thorac Surg 2014;18(2):237–9.

19. Gonzalez-Rivas D, Fieira E, De la Torre M, et al. Bronchovascular right upper lobe reconstruction by uniportal video-assisted thoracoscopic surgery. J Thorac Dis 2014;6(6):861–3.

20. Gonzalez-Rivas D, Delgado M, Fieira E, et al. Single-port video-assisted thoracoscopic lobectomy with pulmonary artery reconstruction. Interact Cardiovasc Thorac Surg 2013;17:889–91.

21. Gonzalez-Rivas D, Delgado M, Fieira E, et al. Double sleeve uniportal video-assisted thoracoscopic lobectomy for non-small cell lung cancer. Ann Cardiothorac Surg 2014;3(2):E2.

22. Huang J, Li J, Qiu Y, et al. Thoracoscopic double sleeve lobectomy in 13 patients: a series report from multi-centers. J Thorac Dis 2015;7(5):834–42.

23. Gonzalez-Rivas D. Uniportal VATS lobectomy and segmentectomy: morbidity and long term results. Presented at European Lung Cancer Conference. Geneva, April 15, 2015.

24. Chung JH, Choi YS, Cho JH, et al. Uniportal video-assisted thoracoscopic lobectomy: an alternative to conventional thoracoscopic lobectomy in lung cancer surgery? Interact Cardiovasc Thorac Surg 2015;20(6):813–9.

25. Lau RW, Ng CS, Kwok MW, et al. Early outcomes following uniportal video-assisted thoracic surgery lung resection. Chest 2014;145(3 Suppl):50A.

26. Gonzalez D, De la Torre M, Paradela M, et al. Video-assisted thoracic surgery lobectomy: 3-year initial experience with 200 cases. Eur J Cardiothorac Surg 2011;40(1):e21–8.

27. Yang Y, Bao F, He Z, et al. Single-port video-assisted thoracoscopic right upper lobectomy using a flexible videoscope. Eur J Cardiothorac Surg 2014;46:496–7.

28. Guo C, Liu C, Lin F, et al. Intrathoracic vertical overhanging approach for placement of an endo-stapler during single-port video-assisted thoracoscopic lobectomy. Eur J Cardiothorac Surg 2016;49:i84–6.

29. Anile M, Diso D, De Giacomo T, et al. Uniportal thoracoscopic lobectomy. Ann Thorac Surg 2013;96(2):745.

30. Guido W, Gonzalez-Rivas D, Duang L, et al. Uniportal video-assisted thoracoscopic right upper sleeve lobectomy. J Visualized Surg 2015;1:10.

31. Gonzalez-Rivas D, Stupnik T, Fernandez R, et al. Intraoperative bleeding control by uniportal video-assisted thoracoscopic surgery. Eur J Cardiothorac Surg 2016;49:i17–24.

32. Delgado Roel M, Fieira Costa EM, González-Rivas D, et al. Uniportal video-assisted thoracoscopic lymph node dissection. J Thorac Dis 2014;6(S6):S665–8.

33. Fernández Prado R, Fieira Costa E, Delgado Roel M, et al. Management of complications by uniportal video-assisted thoracoscopic surgery. J Thorac Dis 2014;6(S6):S669–73.

34. Chen KC, Cheng YJ, Hung MH, et al. Nonintubated thoracoscopic lung resection: a 3-year experience with 285 cases in a single institution. J Thorac Dis 2012;4:347–51.

35. Pompeo E, Mineo TC. Awake operative videothoracoscopic pulmonary resections. Thorac Surg Clin 2008;18:311–20.

36. Chen KC, Cheng YJ, Heng MH, et al. Non-intubated thoracoscopic surgery using regional anesthesia and vagal block and targeted sedation. J Thorac Dis 2014;6(1):31–6.

37. Dong Q, Liang L, Li Y, et al. Anesthesia with nontracheal intubation in thoracic surgery. J Thorac Dis 2012;4:126–30.

38. Gonzalez-Rivas D, Fernandez R, de la Torre M, et al. Single-port thoracoscopic lobectomy in a nonintubated patient: the least invasive procedure for major lung resection? Interact Cardiovasc Thorac Surg 2014;19(4):552–5.

39. Gonzalez-Rivas D, Fernandez R. Single port video-assisted thoracoscopic lobectomy under spontaneous ventilation in a high risk patient. CTSNET; 2014. Available at: http://www.ctsnet.org/article/single-port-video-assisted-thoracoscopic-lobectomy-under-spontaneous-ventilation-high-risk. Accessed November 18, 2014.

40. Gonzalez-Rivas D, Bonome C, Fieira E, et al. Non-intubated video-assisted thoracoscopic lung resections: the future of thoracic surgery? Eur J Cardiothorac Surg 2015. http://dx.doi.org/10.1093/ejcts/ezv136.

41. Gonzalez-Rivas D, De la Torre M, Fernandez R, et al. Uniportal video-assisted thoracoscopic left upper lobectomy under spontaneous ventilation. J Thorac Dis 2015;7(3):494–5.

42. Bertolaccini L, Rocco G, Viti A, et al. Geometrical characteristics of uniportal VATS. J Thorac Dis 2013;5(S3):S214–6.

43. Bertolaccini L, Viti A, Terzi A. Ergon-trial: ergonomic evaluation of single-port access versus three-port access video-assisted thoracic surgery. Surg Endosc 2015;29(10):2934–40.

44. Gonzalez-Rivas D, Yang Y, Sputnik T, et al. Uniportal video-assisted thoracoscopic sleeve resections. Eur J Cardiothorac Surg 2016;49(Suppl 1):i6–16.

45. Nakagawa T, Chiba N, Ueda Y, et al. Clinical experience of sleeve lobectomy with bronchoplasty using a continuous absorbable barbed suture. Gen Thorac Cardiovasc Surg 2015;63(11):640–3.

46. Bagan P, Le Pimpec-Barthes F, Badia A, et al. Bronchial sleeve resections: lung function resurrecting procedure. Eur J Cardiothorac Surg 2008;34:484–7.

47. Xu X, Chen H, Yin W, et al. Thoracoscopic half carina resection and bronchial sleeve resection for central lung cancer. Surg Innov 2014;21(5):481–6.

48. Weder W, Inci I. Carinal resection and sleeve pneumonectomy. Thorac Surg Clin 2014;24(1):77–83.

49. Watanabe Y, Murakami S, Iwa T, et al. The clinical value of high-frequency jet ventilation in major airway reconstructive surgery. Scand J Thorac Cardiovasc Surg 1988;22(3):227–33.

50. Nan YY, Chu Y, Wu YC, et al. Subxiphoid video-assisted thoracoscopic surgery versus standard video-assisted thoracoscopic surgery for anatomic pulmonary lobectomy. J Surg Res 2015;200(1):324–31.

51. Liu CC. First report—20131209 Subxiphoid single port VAT. Available at: http://www.youtube.com/watch?v=Hi_gn8s0VzU. Accessed January 21, 2015.

52. Ng CSH, Wong RHL, Lau RWH, et al. Minimizing chest wall trauma in single port video-assisted thoracic surgery. J Thorac Cardiovasc Surg 2014;147(3):1095–6.

53. Ng CSH, Wong RHL, Lau RWH, et al. Single port video-assisted thoracic surgery: advancing scope technology. Eur J Cardiothorac Surg 2015;47(4):751.

54. Ng CSH. Uniportal video assisted thoracic surgery: a look into the future. Eur J Cardiothorac Surg 2015;49:i1–2.

55. Ng CSH, Gonzalez Rivas D, D'Amico T, et al. Uniportal VATS: a new era in lung cancer surgery. J Thorac Dis 2015;7(8):1489–91.

56. Lardinois D, Ris HB. Minimally invasive video-endoscopic sympathectomy by use of a transaxillary single port approach. Eur J Cardiothorac Surg 2002;21:67–70.

57. Ng CSH, Yeung ECL, Wong RHL, et al. Single-port sympathectomy for palmar hyperhidrosis with Vasoview® HemoPro 2 endoscopic vein harvesting device. J Thorac Cardiovasc Surg 2012;144:1256–7.

58. Ng CSH. Uniportal VATS in Asia. J Thorac Dis 2013;5(S3):S221–5.

59. Lazarus J. The airscope: a novel wireless laparoscope. J Med Devices 2012;6:044501–3.

60. Ng CSH, Rocco G, Wong RHL, et al. Uniportal and single incision video assisted thoracic surgery: the state of the art. Interact Cardiovasc Thorac Surg 2014;19(4):661–6.

61. Ng CSH, Pickens A, Siegel JM, et al. A novel narrow profile articulating powered vascular stapler provides superior access and hemostasis equivalent to conventional devices. Eur J Cardiothorac Surg 2016;49:i73–8.

62. Oh Y, Lee YS, Quan YH, et al. Thoracoscopic color and fluorescence imaging system for sentinel lymph node mapping in porcine lung using indocyanine green-neomannosyl human serum albumin: intraoperative image-guided sentinel nodes navigation. Ann Surg Oncol 2014;21(4):1182–8.

63. Ng CSH. Single port thoracic surgery: a new direction. Korean J Thorac Cardiovasc Surg 2014;47(4):327–32.

64. Khereba M, Thiffault V, Goudie E, et al. Transtracheal thoracic natural orifice transluminal endoscopic

surgery (NOTES) in a swine model. Surg Endosc 2015. [Epub ahead of print].

65. Zhu LH, Chen L, Yang S, et al. Embryonic NOTES thoracic sympathectomy for palmar hyperhidrosis: results of a novel technique and comparison with the conventional VATS procedure. Surg Endosc 2013;27:4124–9.

66. Zhu LH, Du Q, Chen L, et al. One-year followup period after transumbilical thoracic sympathectomy for hyperhidrosis: outcomes and consequences. J Thorac Cardiovasc Surg 2014; 147:25–8.

67. Wu YC, Yen-Chu, Yeh CJ, et al. Feasibility of transumbilical surgical lung biopsy and pericardial window creation. Surg Innov 2014;21(1):15–21.

68. Santos BF, Hungness ES. Natural orifice translumenal endoscopic surgery: progress in humans since white paper. World J Gastroenterol 2011;17(13):1655–65.

69. Simaan N, Bajo A, Reiter A, et al. Lessons learned using the IREP for single-port access surgery. J Robot Surg 2013;7:235–40.

Electromagnetic Navigational Bronchoscopy for Peripheral Pulmonary Nodules

Satish Kalanjeri, MD, MRCP[a],*, Thomas R. Gildea, MD, MS[b]

KEYWORDS

- Peripheral pulmonary nodules • Electromagnetic navigational bronchoscopy • ENB
- Lung cancer • Solitary pulmonary nodule

KEY POINTS

- Electromagnetic navigational bronchoscopy (ENB) is a useful addition to the array of modalities available to sample peripheral lung lesions.
- ENB's utility in diagnosing peripheral lesions has been steadily increasing since the Food and Drug Administration first approved it in 2004.
- ENB offers an opportunity to venture into therapeutic interventions in peripheral lung nodules, a prospect that has remained elusive to bronchoscopists for a long time.
- Better identification of predictors of success with ENB, superior safety profile, and ability to performed staging endobronchial ultrasound at the same time have made ENB the preferred modality in the management of peripheral lung nodules.

INTRODUCTION

Peripheral pulmonary nodules have long been a diagnostic challenge for pulmonologists. Unlike endobronchial lesions, lack of direct visualization of a peripheral nodule during bronchoscopy and inability to guide the bronchoscope or instruments accurately through the smaller airways leading to the lesion sets it up for unsatisfactory sampling, resulting in poor diagnostic yield. Conventional bronchoscopy and transbronchial biopsies have a very low sensitivity (14%–63%) for diagnosing malignant lesions.[1,2] The yield is particularly low (30%) for lesions less than 2 cm in diameter.[1,2] With the introduction of lung cancer screening with low-dose computed tomography (CT), pulmonologists are expected to deal with peripheral lung nodules more than ever before. The National Lung Cancer Screening Trial demonstrated lung nodules in at least 39% of the participants, of which 72% required further investigation.[3] Although CT-guided transthoracic needle biopsy of peripheral lung nodules has a high sensitivity for malignant lesions (up to 90%), it is fraught with moderately high complication rates, up to 24% in some studies.[4] Therefore, refining bronchoscopic techniques may offer safer ways to sample these nodules and perhaps add additional techniques to acquire more tissue and perform a more comprehensive evaluation, including mediastinal staging when appropriate. With the advent of endobronchial ultrasound (EBUS), a single bronchoscopic procedure offers the ability to sample the nodule as well as mediastinal and hilar lymph nodes, effectively offering diagnosis and staging in a single sitting.

[a] Interventional Pulmonology, Section of Pulmonary, Critical Care & Sleep Medicine, Louisiana State University Health Sciences Center, Shreveport, LA 71130, USA; [b] Section of Bronchology, Respiratory Institute, Cleveland Clinic Foundation, Cleveland, OH 44195, USA
* Corresponding author.
E-mail address: skala1@lsuhsc.edu

Thorac Surg Clin 26 (2016) 203–213
http://dx.doi.org/10.1016/j.thorsurg.2015.12.008
1547-4127/16/$ – see front matter © 2016 Elsevier Inc. All rights reserved.

Navigational bronchoscopy is one tool among several designed to address part of this clinical need. There are now several different navigation systems that are available. Each technology uses images from the CT scan to reconstruct a 3-dimensional (3D) map of the airways, thereby creating a virtual bronchoscopy with a broncho-scopic view and pathway via the airway lumen. Although this is an exciting invention, it does little to actually guide instruments to the peripheral lung lesions. Addition of electromagnetic (EM) tracking to virtual bronchoscopy has allowed real-time positional guidance and directional cues. Bronchoscopists may then use these virtual road maps to guide sampling instruments to the peripheral nodule, just like the global positioning system.

The most widely used EM navigational bron-choscopy (ENB) system is the superDimension system currently owned by Medtronic (Minneapo-lis, MN) and the newer system the Veran Thoracic Navigation System (Veran Medical Technologies Inc, St Louis, MO).

ELECTROMAGNETIC NAVIGATIONAL BRONCHOSCOPY

Earlier predecessors of the currently available sys-tems incorporated the 3 basic components of the technology. There is a need for multiplanar CT reconstruction, a positional sensor, and a mag-netic field generator. One of the earliest examples was a 3D EM tracking system and published by Solomon and colleagues[5] using a porcine model and later Hautmann and colleagues[6] used a similar system for peripheral lesions and described the basic components.

The current superDimension system now in version 7 has the same basic components but more advanced planning software and naviga-tional tools.

In order to achieve this, the system consists of the following steps or phases:

1. Planning phase (reconstruction of CT scan and creation of a virtual road map to a defined target)
2. Registration phase (creation of EM field around patients, and synchronizing sensors overlap the virtual and actual patient anatomy)
3. Navigation phase (using the positional infor-mation to guide instruments to the target lesion)

The Veran system is similar but allows a process to skip registration if the CT is obtained with the dedicated skin sensor on the chest.

PLANNING PHASE

The planning phase requires dedicated system software. The format of the CT images is loaded into system. The recommended CT scan specifi-cations are slightly different for each system and scanner: The primary important aspect to know is that the scans tend to be a higher dose of radi-ation with higher resolution and image overlap in the reconstructions. You can refer to the manufac-turer recommendations for each navigation sys-tem and CT scanner specifications.

Once the CT data are successfully imported, there are several steps to complete the planning. The screen will generally show multiplanar CT re-constructions (axial, coronal, and sagittal planes) and some other image reconstruction with stan-dard tool bars for interacting with the software (**Fig. 1**). The images are scrolled to reveal the target lesion (see **Fig. 1**). The target lesion is then marked as the navigation end point. Using one or more views, the crosshair on the lesion can be adjusted to define the size and dimension of the lesion (**Fig. 2**). Then the operator completes the steps of linking the lesion to an appropriate airway. During this process, the software automatically creates a pathway from the trachea to the target. The pathway is reviewed and accepted as is or modified according to the operator's satisfaction. This part of the procedure requires some expertise to understand airway and lesion relationships and adjust pathways to see if unrealistic acute angles from the closest airway to the lesion would nega-tively impact the ability to obtain samples. Once target acquisition is complete, a virtual fly-through can be performed to help with the bron-choscopic portion of the navigation (**Fig. 3**).

The next step is to identify registration points in case a manual registration needs to be performed during the procedure (superDimension). The soft-ware asks the operator to identify points on the vir-tual bronchoscopy that can be easily identified during the real-time bronchoscopy procedure. These points include the main carina, right upper lobe, right middle lobe, left upper lobe, and left lower lobe (**Fig. 4**). Once planning is completed, the data are saved first and then can be exported to a USB, which is then loaded to the procedure station.

Based on the planning, the choice of superDi-mension Edge Catheter or Veran tip-tracked or bi-opsy tools will be selected.

PROCEDURE REGISTRATION

After a standard airway examination is done and there is still a need to perform the navigational pro-cedure, the instrumentation is set up to do

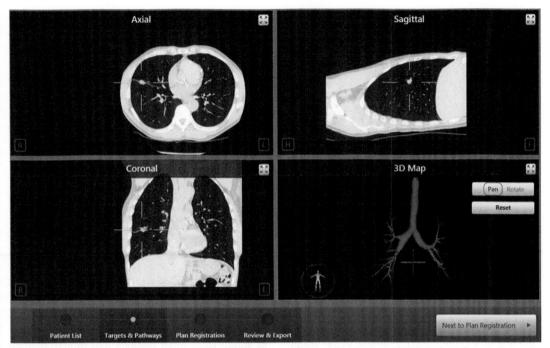

Fig. 1. Planning phase - Multiplanar views of the target lesion.

registration. It must be checked that a therapeutic bronchoscope with 2.8-mm working channel is used; or in the case of the Veran system, the guidance tool or the tip-tracked instrument set must be prepared.

AUTOMATIC REGISTRATION

During this process, the sensor or locatable guide (LG) passively makes hundreds of positional and

matches this to the volume of the virtual 3D tracheobronchial tree. To ensure accuracy, the bronchoscope should be advanced an equal distance into each lobar bronchus. Once the software has enough data points to create an accurate registration, a virtual bronchoscopic image will appear on the screen. At this point the scope is withdrawn and stationed at the main carina. The virtual bronchoscopic image should be manually adjusted on the screen to match the orientation

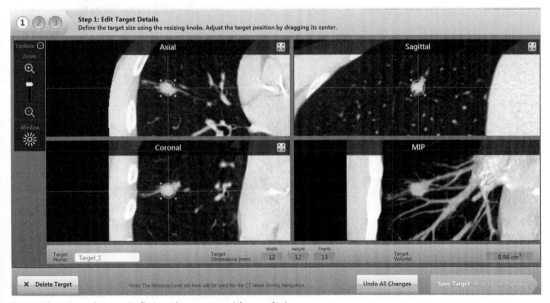

Fig. 2. Planning phase - Defining the target with crosshairs.

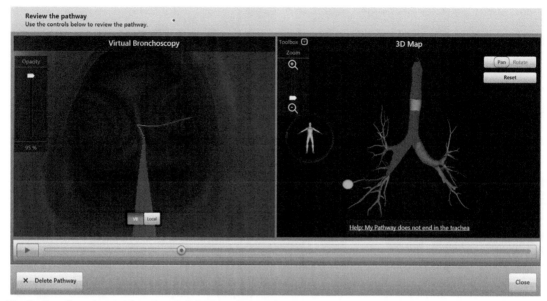

Fig. 3. Planning phase - Virtual path ('Fly through') to the target.

of the real-time bronchoscopic image. In the Veran system this would be a manual registration whereby this step can be skipped if the sensors are already in place when the CT is performed.

MANUAL REGISTRATION

Occasionally the automatic registration process described earlier cannot be completed because of anatomic or other glitches that require manual registration to be performed. The manual registration requires manual identification of the registration points saved during the planning phase. To achieve this, onscreen instructions are followed and the LG is placed serially on preset registration points identified and saved during the planning process. This process should include at least 5 registration points, one of the points being the

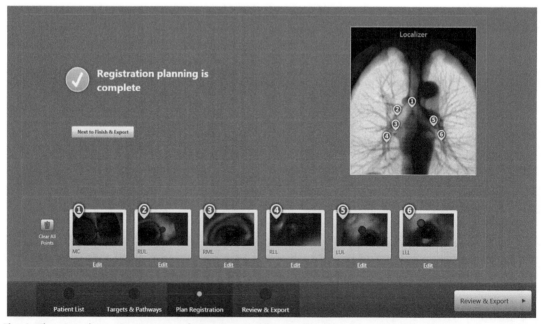

Fig. 4. Planning phase - Registration of prominent landmarks ('Registration points') in case manual registration has to be performed during the procedure.

main carina and 2 in each lower lobe bronchi. Because this is not a dynamic process, the registration algorithm will incur variable CT to body error also known as average fiducial target registration error (AFTRE). This error used to be reported and displayed by the software after the registration is completed. If the AFTRE score is acceptable (<5 mm), the operator will accept the registration. If the AFTRE score is not acceptable, the manual registration process can be restarted. Once the registration is completed, the navigation procedure can be commenced. The AFTRE is a measure of how much different the probe may be in the virtual world from actual patients. This measure is a sphere of uncertainty and cannot be visually corrected in most cases, but obvious errors may be seen with the qualitative check as described earlier. Through the course of the procedure the computer can make additional adjustment to align virtual and actual anatomic locations.

NAVIGATION PHASE

Because the actual execution of the navigation in each system is different, the authors focus specifically on the superDimension system because they have no clinical experience with the Veran system.

The bronchoscope is wedged into the subsegment leading to the target lesion. The EWC and LG are then slowly advanced toward the lesion. This advancement is achieved by rotating and advancing the LG along the purple pathway generated on virtual bronchoscopy images. The LG can be directed with rotation of the edge catheter along the pathway. The target lesion is represented as a green sphere on all of the system view ports. As the LG gets closer to the lesion, the green dot seems to get larger (**Fig. 5**). The distance between the LG tip and the target lesion is displayed onscreen (see **Fig. 5**). Once the LG reaches the desired location close to the target, the EWC or edge catheter is fixed at the proximal end of the biopsy channel of the bronchoscope by a locking mechanism and the LG is withdrawn (EWC is left in place). Fluoroscopy can be used to confirm the LG position before it is removed. Once the LG is removed (**Fig. 6**), real-time confirmation of the target lesion may be attempted by use of radial probe endobronchial ultrasound or confocal endomicroscopy. Various sampling instruments can then be used to obtain tissue. The LG projects a considerable distance at the proximal end of the catheter and even further from the bronchoscope. Therefore, any instrumentation that is used should have considerable length to traverse through the bronchoscope to the target lesion. It is advisable to perform marking on the instruments if fluoroscopy is not used. The use of fluoroscopy is not mandatory but has been quite helpful in the authors' practice when it comes to biopsy technique.

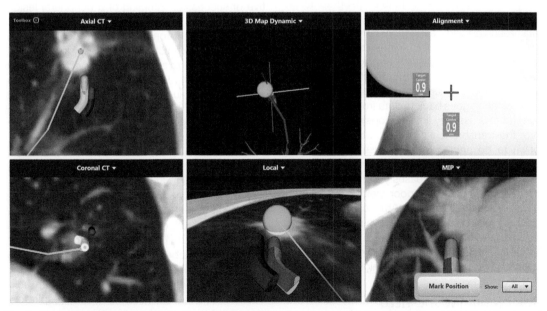

Fig. 5. Navigation phase - Multiplanar views of the virtual images as the locator guide approaches the target lesion. Please note the green dot that is marked over the target lesion and is shown to be 9 mm from the locator guide tip.

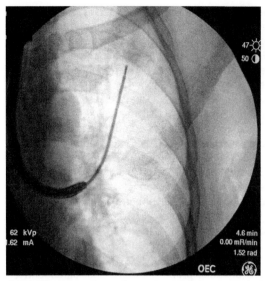

Fig. 6. Fluoroscopic conformation of locator guided near the target lesion.

BIOPSY TECHNIQUE

Interestingly, little has been written about this in the literature and yet is a critical part of the ability to obtain diagnostic tissue. The ability to use all standard biopsy instruments is one of the main advantages of using a catheter-based technology. In this way, understanding and using biopsy instrumentation to overcome several airway-to-lesion variations and achieve a yield is critical. In many articles there were limits on the type of instruments used, and many of these tend to be geographic. In Europe and Asia, there is little use of peripheral transbronchial needle aspiration (TBNA) techniques when ENB is performed; but these have been shown to be associated with the highest yields in the prenavigation era,[7] and the idea that multiple biopsy tools are complementary and should be used in combination goes back to data from 1976.[8,9] Yet many articles use very limited biopsy techniques in favor the transbronchial biopsy, which has been shown to be one of the least useful tools even compared with simple suction aspiration; but each when used together increases yield.[10,11] The most recent article describing poor yield in peripheral lesions published from the American College of Chest Physicians Quality Improvement Registry, Evaluation, and Education (AQuIRE) registry noted that peripheral TBNA was used in only 16.4% of cases but was associated with a higher yield.[12]

DATA ON DIAGNOSTIC YIELD

Table 1 shows major studies with ENB, the diagnostic yield, and other characteristics, including lesion size, number of lesions, registration error, and pneumothorax rates. These studies vary widely in their design, sample size, and end points. Besides prevalence of nonmalignant conditions, such as histoplasmosis, in study population may also affect ENBs sensitivity for diagnosis of malignant peripheral nodules.

In a meta-analysis of 39 studies using guided bronchoscopy for diagnosis of peripheral lung lesion, 10 studies used virtual bronchoscopy only and 11 studies used ENB.[13] Interestingly, the diagnostic yield for virtual bronchoscopy without ENB was higher (72%) than ENB (67%). The reason for this slightly lower yield is unclear despite the fact that ENB has a virtual bronchoscopy component.

A more recent meta-analysis of 16 studies using ENB technology for diagnosis of peripheral lung lesions showed diagnostic yields ranging from 56.0% to 87.5%.[14] The pooled diagnostic yield was 64.9%, whereas sensitivity to detect malignancy was 71.0%. The negative predictive value for detection of lung cancer was 52%.

Most studies show that successful navigation to the target area occurs in more than 90% of occasions. However, there remains a discrepancy between successful navigation and successful sampling. Respiratory motion and registration errors may play a role in this discrepancy.

PREDICTORS FOR SUCCESS

Several factors have been recognized as predictive of successful sampling of a peripheral lesion using ENB.

Presence of a bronchus to the lesion seems to be a strong predictor of successful sampling. The impact of the so-called air bronchus sign on CT scan was studied in 51 consecutive patients with peripheral lung nodules with a mean lesion size of 25 mm.[15] The overall diagnostic yield was 67%; but for lesions with the air bronchus sign, it was 88%.

Lobar location of the nodule seems to play a role too. However, the inference is variable between studies. In one study the diagnostic yield from lesions located in the upper lobes was 77%, whereas it was 29% if the lesions were located in the lower lobes[16]; other studies have not noticed this difference.[17,18] The lower yield from lower lobe lesions has been attributed to diaphragmatic movement resulting in navigation error as the CT images are obtained during a single breath hold and does not take into account respiratory movement.

There are conflicting data regarding the size of lesions as a determinant of diagnostic yield with

Table 1
ENB: diagnostic yield and other characteristics

Study, Year	Technology	Anesthesia	Mean Size (mm)	AFTRE (mm)	No. PPL	Diagnostic Yield (%)	PTX (%)
Becker et al,[37] 2005	ENB, Fluoro	GA	39.8	6.2	29	69	3.3
Hautmann et al,[6] 2005	ENB, Fluoro	CS	22	NA	16	66	0
Gildea et al,[17] 2006	ENB, Fluoro	CS	22.8	6.6	58	74	3.4
Schwarz et al,[38] 2006	ENB, Fluoro	CS	33.5	NA	13	69	0
Markis et al,[24] 2007	ENB	GA/CS	23.5	8.7	40	62.5	7.5
Eberhardt et al,[19] 2007	ENB	GA/CS	24	4.6	93	67	2.2
Wilson and Bartlett,[18] 2007	ENB, Fluoro, OSE	CS	21	4	222	60	1.2
Eberhardt et al,[16] 2007	ENB	GA/CS	26	NA	39	74	6
Lamprecht et al,[39] 2009	ENB, PET-CT, ROSE	GA	30	3.9	13	77	0
Bertoletti et al,[40] 2009	ENB	Nitrous oxide	31	4.7	53	77	4
Seijo et al,[15] 2010	ENB, ROSE	CS	25	4	51	66.7	0
Eberhardt et al,[10] 2010	ENB, RP-EBUS	GA/CS	23.3	3.6	54	75.5	1.9
Mahajan et al,[41] 2011	ENB, Fluoro	CS	20	NA	49	77	10
Lamprecht et al,[20] 2012	ENB, PET-CT, ROSE	GA	27	NA	112	84	1.8
Pearlstein et al,[42] 2012	ENB, ROSE	GA	28	4	101	85	5.8
Karnak et al,[22] 2013	ENB, ROSE	CS	23	4.4	35	91	3.9
Loo et al,[43] 2014	ENB, PET-CT, ROSE	GA	26	NA	50	94	0

Abbreviations: CS, conscious sedation; Fluoro, fluoroscopy; GA, general anesthesia; NA, not available; PPL, peripheral pulmonary lesion; PTX, pneumothorax; ROSE, rapid onsite cytologic evaluation; RP, radial probe.
Data from Refs.[6,10,15–20,22,24,37–43]

ENB. Lesions less than 3 cm had a diagnostic yield of 72%, whereas the yield was 82% for lesions greater than 3 cm in one of the first prospective studies with ENB.[17] However, some of the larger subsequent studies noted the diagnostic yield to be independent of lesion size.[16,19]

The learning curve with the technology also seems to play a role in determining diagnostic yield. The diagnostic yield in one study was noted to increase from 80.0% to 87.5% after 30 to 40 ENB procedures.[20] In an earlier study of the first 48 ENB procedures that were performed at their institution, the patients were categorized into groups A, B, or C based on the chronologic time they had their procedure.[21] The diagnostic yield in group A (early cases) was 57.8% and significantly lower than later cases (groups B and C 87.5% and 93.3%, respectively).

The AFTRE may affect sampling success. The AFTRE is difference in the location of the tip of the locator guide in actual patients compared with where it is expected to be on the virtual 3D airway map created from the CT images on the software. AFTRE less than 5 mm has been attributed to better yields.[18,22]

The ideal type of anesthesia for ENB has remained a controversial topic. Pooled data from previous studies favor general anesthesia (diagnostic yield 69%) over conscious sedation (diagnostic yield 57%).[14] These studies are mostly retrospective and do not make a head-to-head comparison. However, a recent retrospective analysis of 120 lesions compared the effect of general anesthesia versus conscious sedation for diagnostic yield; this study did not demonstrate significant difference in diagnostic yields between the two modes of anesthesia.[23] Most experts, however, seem to agree that procedural time and patient comfort are better with general anesthesia than conscious sedation.

Finally, some operators are simply not very good at navigational bronchoscopy. In the Makris and colleagues'[24] study operator A never achieved a yield of greater than 42.8% over 14 cases, whereas operator B performed 26 procedures and had a yield that decreased from 76.9% to 69.2% from the first 13 to second 13 cases.[24]

ELECTROMAGNETIC NAVIGATIONAL BRONCHOSCOPY AND THE ROLE OF RAPID ONSITE CYTOPATHOLOGIC EVALUATION

Rapid onsite cytopathologic evaluation (ROSE) has been studied as a factor affecting the diagnostic yield of ENB. A study of 112 consecutive patients to undergo ENB for peripheral lesions evaluated the effect of PET-CT before the procedure and ROSE during the ENB on the overall diagnostic yield.[20] The study found diagnostic yields of 75.6% and 89.6% for lesions less than 2 cm and greater than 2 cm, respectively. The overall diagnostic yield was 83.9%, and this higher yield was attributed to the combination of PET and ROSE being used to aid ENB.

Another study of ENB on 35 consecutive patients with peripheral lesions used ROSE to aid the procedure and found a diagnostic yield of 91% with ENB and ROSE for peripheral lesions (mean size 23 mm).[22] The investigators found that the average number of passes required was only 3 for each of the lesion while using ROSE.

Although these studies provide encouraging data, lack of controls and an unusually high diagnostic yield compared with other centers that use ROSE suggest that ROSE, although useful, may not be the strongest predictor of improved diagnostic yield with ENB.

A recent meta-analysis, however, did show a pooled sensitivity of 80.2% from 4 studies using ROSE, whereas pooled sensitivity of ENB from 10 studies that did not use ROSE was 66.3%.[14] However, the discrepancy in the number of studies included for each arm does now allow us to draw definitive conclusions.

One of the primary problems with using historical data with new technology is the constant evolution of the technique over time. Meta-analysis is a classic example whereby the mean outcome may have nothing to do with the most current version of the procedure and it does not account for new biopsy tools or operator skill over time. Changes in practice like anesthesia type, CT resolution, software version, and clinical judgment

have been introduced; to not account for major differences like these over time cannot be adequately ascertained. There is no doubt some people have never achieved clinical competence and others have expertise, and the authors have many debates about the unknowns of patient selection and other cognitive biases.

THERAPEUTIC APPLICATIONS OF ELECTROMAGNETIC NAVIGATIONAL BRONCHOSCOPY

Stereotactic radiosurgery has gained in clinical utility over time. Patients who are deemed medically inoperable may derive equivalent benefit from stereotactic radiosurgery as patients who undergo surgical resection.[25] Fiducial markers placed in the tumor or in close proximity allow for exact localization of the lesion during stereotactic radiosurgery for some delivery systems. Traditionally fiducial placement with CT guidance has a pneumothorax rate as high as 33%.[26] Bronchoscopic fiducial placement offers a safer and reliable approach.[27,28] The reliability of the bronchoscopic approach seems to be tied to the type of fiducial used. In a study of 52 consecutive patients who underwent ENB for fiducial marker placement, 4 patients received a total of 17 linear markers, whereas 49 patients received a total of 217 coil-spring markers. A total of 215 (99%) coil-spring markers and 8 (47%) linear markers were noted to still be in place at the time of stereotactic radiosurgery planning.[29]

Another therapeutic application of ENB-directed fiducial marker placement is in patients who can undergo wedge resection but not lobectomy. Placement of a fiducial marker or even injection of a dye marker using ENB can help localize the target area during surgery.[30,31] This practice has allowed patients with prior pneumonectomy to undergo wedge resection in the remaining lung.

BRACHYTHERAPY

Brachytherapy of small tumors for patients deemed inoperable is an option particularly if radiosurgery is not available. There is a reported case of a right upper lobe tumor that was successfully navigated to by ENB and a brachytherapy catheter advance into the tumor. Radiographic follow-up of the patient revealed remission of the tumor.[32] A case series of 18 patients with peripheral tumors who were treated with ENB was also presented at a conference with relatively favorable outcomes (50% remission).[33]

Soon we will have opportunities to evaluate ablative techniques not yet approved by the

Food and Drug Administration (FDA) approved. Microwave ablation seems to be closest to clinical trials based on predictable treatment characteristics of the device absent any clinical data.

TISSUE ADEQUACY FOR MOLECULAR MARKERS

Molecular profiling has become the routine practice in non–small cell lung cancer (NSCLC), specifically adenocarcinomas. Cytologic samples have been shown to be reliable in determining epidermal growth factor receptor (EGFR), anaplastic lymphoma kinase (ALK), and K-ras mutations in patients with NSCLC.[34] Samples obtained from peripheral lung nodules via ENB have also shown to be adequate for reliable mutational analysis. A retrospective analysis of samples obtained from 65 cases of NSCLC diagnosed by ENB demonstrated successful histologic subtyping in 100% of the cases.[35] Of the 16 cases that underwent surgical resection, the concordance rate for histologic subtyping was 87.7%. Fifteen samples were sent for EGFR and 2 samples for ALK mutational analysis. Fourteen of 15 samples (93.3%) were deemed adequate for EGFR analysis, and both the samples sent for ALK mutational analysis were considered adequate.

SAFETY

ENB and all bronchoscopic techniques have a significantly better safety profile compared with transthoracic needle aspiration of peripheral lung nodules. The rate of pneumothorax is particularly low (0%–10%), and a major reason is ENB allows for nodule sampling without puncturing pleural surfaces. Even in patients with emphysematous lung, ENB is considered safe. In a meta-analysis of 1033 procedures, pneumothorax was noted in 32 patients (3.1%), of which only 17 patients (1.6%) required chest tube placement.[14]

Bleeding requiring no specific intervention was noted in 0.9% of cases. Self-limited hematoma has also been reported.[14] A reason for rarity with bleeding complications may be the use of the EWC that creates a tamponade effect in the smaller airways.

Because ENB operates by creation of an EM field, there are concerns about its safety in the presence of permanent pacemakers and cardiac defibrillators. This concern was addressed in a study of 24 patients with pacemakers and defibrillators who underwent ENB.[36] The pacemakers were interrogated before the procedure, and ENB was performed in the presence of an electrophysiology and a programmer. All 24 cases were successfully performed without arrhythmic events or device dysfunction. Additionally, the investigators noted no artifact or registration errors due to the presence of these devices. Their diagnostic yield of 75% was in keeping with their prior results and that noted in literature.

SUMMARY

ENB is a useful addition to the array of modalities available to sample peripheral lung lesions. Its utility in diagnosing peripheral lesions has been steadily increasing since the FDA first approved it in 2004. The improvement can be attributed to continuous refinement in technology, increasing training and experience with the procedure, perhaps widespread availability of ROSE, and better patient selection. It may also be attributable to improvements of the technology and more available tools to perform biopsy of the peripheral lung, but also the improvement of cytopathology and immunohistochemistry experience is working with small biopsies. Successful navigation to the target lesion is achieved almost all the time, but the diagnostic accuracy does not exceed 74%[14] suggesting problems with biopsy technique rather than navigation in many cases. The negative predictive value for malignant lesions remains low, as will all sampling techniques. Routine use of real-time confirmation of target lesion after successful navigation using radial probe EBUS or con-focal endomicroscopy, and further improvement in technology may improve diagnostic outcomes with ENB in the future but are currently adjuncts that predict improved yield rather than directly improving it. Furthermore, ENB offers an opportunity to venture into therapeutic interventions in peripheral lung nodules, a prospect that has remained elusive to bronchoscopists for a long time. Better identification of predictors of success with ENB, superior safety profile, and ability to perform staging EBUS at the same time have made ENB the preferred modality in the management of peripheral lung nodules.

REFERENCES

1. Popovich J Jr, Kvale PA, Eichenhorn MS, et al. Diagnostic accuracy of multiple biopsies from flexible fiberoptic bronchoscopy. A comparison of central versus peripheral carcinoma. Am Rev Respir Dis 1982;125(5):521–3.
2. Rivera MP, Mehta AC, American College of Chest Physicians. Initial diagnosis of lung cancer: ACCP evidence-based clinical practice guidelines (2nd edition). Chest 2007;132(3 Suppl):131S–48S.

3. National Lung Screening Trial Research Team, Aberle DR, Adams AM, et al. Reduced lung-cancer mortality with low-dose computed tomographic screening. N Engl J Med 2011;365(5):395–409.

4. Wiener RS, Schwartz LM, Woloshin S, et al. Population-based risk for complications after transthoracic needle lung biopsy of a pulmonary nodule: an analysis of discharge records. Ann Intern Med 2011; 155(3):137–44.

5. Solomon SB, White P Jr, Acker DE, et al. Real-time bronchoscope tip localization enables three-dimensional CT image guidance for transbronchial needle aspiration in swine. Chest 1998;114(5): 1405–10.

6. Hautmann H, Schneider A, Pinkau T, et al. Electromagnetic catheter navigation during bronchoscopy: validation of a novel method by conventional fluoroscopy. Chest 2005;128(1):382–7.

7. Schreiber G, McCrory DC. Performance characteristics of different modalities for diagnosis of suspected lung cancer: summary of published evidence. Chest 2003;123(1 Suppl):115S–28S.

8. Kvale PA, Bode FR, Kini S. Diagnostic accuracy in lung cancer; comparison of techniques used in association with flexible fiberoptic bronchoscopy. Chest 1976;69(6):752–7.

9. Odronic SI, Gildea TR, Chute DJ. Electromagnetic navigation bronchoscopy-guided fine needle aspiration for the diagnosis of lung lesions. Diagn Cytopathol 2014;42(12):1045–50.

10. Eberhardt R, Morgan RK, Ernst A, et al. Comparison of suction catheter versus forceps biopsy for sampling of solitary pulmonary nodules guided by electromagnetic navigational bronchoscopy. Respiration 2010;79(1):54–60.

11. Franke KJ, Nilius G, Ruhle KH. Transbronchial biopsy in comparison with catheter aspiration in the diagnosis of peripheral pulmonary nodules. Pneumologie 2006;60(1):7–10.

12. Ost DE, Ernst A, Lei X, et al. Diagnostic yield and complications of bronchoscopy for peripheral lung lesions: results of the AQuIRE registry. Am J Respir Crit Care Med 2016;193(1):68–77.

13. Wang Memoli JS, Nietert PJ, Silvestri GA. Meta-analysis of guided bronchoscopy for the evaluation of the pulmonary nodule. Chest 2012;142(2):385–93.

14. Gex G, Pralong JA, Combescure C, et al. Diagnostic yield and safety of electromagnetic navigation bronchoscopy for lung nodules: a systematic review and meta-analysis. Respiration 2014;87(2):165–76.

15. Seijo LM, de Torres JP, Lozano MD, et al. Diagnostic yield of electromagnetic navigation bronchoscopy is highly dependent on the presence of a bronchus sign on CT imaging: results from a prospective study. Chest 2010;138(6):1316–21.

16. Eberhardt R, Anantham D, Ernst A, et al. Multimodality bronchoscopic diagnosis of peripheral lung lesions: a randomized controlled trial. Am J Respir Crit Care Med 2007;176(1):36–41.

17. Gildea TR, Mazzone PJ, Karnak D, et al. Electromagnetic navigation diagnostic bronchoscopy: a prospective study. Am J Respir Crit Care Med 2006;174(9):982–9.

18. Wilson D, Bartlett R. Improved diagnostic yield of bronchoscopy in a community practice: combination of electromagnetic navigation system and rapid on-site evaluation. J Bronchol 2007;14(4):227–32.

19. Eberhardt R, Anantham D, Herth F, et al. Electromagnetic navigation diagnostic bronchoscopy in peripheral lung lesions. Chest 2007;131(6):1800–5.

20. Lamprecht B, Porsch P, Wegleitner B, et al. Electromagnetic navigation bronchoscopy (ENB): increasing diagnostic yield. Respir Med 2012; 106(5):710–5.

21. Bansal S, Hale K, Sethi S, et al. Electromagnetic navigational bronchoscopy: a learning curve analysis. Chest 2007;132(4_MeetingAbstracts):514b.

22. Karnak D, Ciledag A, Ceyhan K, et al. Rapid on-site evaluation and low registration error enhance the success of electromagnetic navigation bronchoscopy. Ann Thorac Med 2013;8(1):28–32.

23. Bowling MR, Kohan MW, Walker P, et al. The effect of general anesthesia versus intravenous sedation on diagnostic yield and success in electromagnetic navigation bronchoscopy. J Bronchology Interv Pulmonol 2015;22(1):5–13.

24. Makris D, Scherpereel A, Leroy S, et al. Electromagnetic navigation diagnostic bronchoscopy for small peripheral lung lesions. Eur Respir J 2007;29(6): 1187–92.

25. Pennathur A, Luketich JD, Heron DE, et al. Stereotactic radiosurgery for the treatment of stage I non-small cell lung cancer in high-risk patients. J Thorac Cardiovasc Surg 2009;137(3):597–604.

26. Yousefi S, Collins BT, Reichner CA, et al. Complications of thoracic computed tomography-guided fiducial placement for the purpose of stereotactic body radiation therapy. Clin Lung Cancer 2007; 8(4):252–6.

27. Harley DP, Krimsky WS, Sarkar S, et al. Fiducial marker placement using endobronchial ultrasound and navigational bronchoscopy for stereotactic radiosurgery: an alternative strategy. Ann Thorac Surg 2010;89(2):368–73 [discussion: 373–4].

28. Anantham D, Feller-Kopman D, Shanmugham LN, et al. Electromagnetic navigation bronchoscopy-guided fiducial placement for robotic stereotactic radiosurgery of lung tumors: a feasibility study. Chest 2007;132(3):930–5.

29. Schroeder C, Hejal R, Linden PA. Coil spring fiducial markers placed safely using navigation bronchoscopy in inoperable patients allows accurate delivery of CyberKnife stereotactic radiosurgery. J Thorac Cardiovasc Surg 2010;140(5):1137–42.

30. Andrade RS. Electromagnetic navigation bronchoscopy-guided thoracoscopic wedge resection of small pulmonary nodules. Semin Thorac Cardiovasc Surg 2010;22(3):262–5.

31. Krimsky WS, Minnich DJ, Cattaneo SM, et al. Thoracoscopic detection of occult indeterminate pulmonary nodules using bronchoscopic pleural dye marking. J Community Hosp Intern Med Perspect 2014;4. http://dx.doi.org/10.3402/jchimp.v4.23084.

32. Harms W, Krempien R, Grehn C, et al. Electromagnetically navigated brachytherapy as a new treatment option for peripheral pulmonary tumors. Strahlenther Onkol 2006;182(2):108–11.

33. Becker HD, McLemore T, Harms W. Electromagnetic navigation and endobronchial ultrasound for brachytherapy of inoperable peripheral lung cancer. Chest 2008;134(S):396.

34. Lozano MD, Zulueta JJ, Echeveste JI, et al. Assessment of epidermal growth factor receptor and K-ras mutation status in cytological stained smears of non-small cell lung cancer patients: correlation with clinical outcomes. Oncologist 2011; 16(6):877–85.

35. Ha D, Choi H, Almeida FA, et al. Histologic and molecular characterization of lung cancer with tissue obtained by electromagnetic navigation bronchoscopy. J Bronchology Interv Pulmonol 2013;20(1): 10–5.

36. Khan AY, Berkowitz D, Krimsky WS, et al. Safety of pacemakers and defibrillators in electromagnetic navigation bronchoscopy. Chest 2013;143(1):75–81.

37. Becker H, Herth F, Ernst A, et al. Bronchoscopic biopsy of peripheral lung lesions under electromagnetic guidance: a pilot study. J Bronchol 2005;12(1):9–13.

38. Schwarz Y, Greif J, Becker HD, et al. Real-time electromagnetic navigation bronchoscopy to peripheral lung lesions using overlaid CT images: the first human study. Chest 2006; 129(4):988–94.

39. Lamprecht B, Porsch P, Pirich C, et al. Electromagnetic navigation bronchoscopy in combination with PET-CT and rapid on-site cytopathologic examination for diagnosis of peripheral lung lesions. Lung 2009;187(1):55–9.

40. Bertoletti L, Robert A, Cottier M, et al. Accuracy and feasibility of electromagnetic navigated bronchoscopy under nitrous oxide sedation for pulmonary peripheral opacities: an outpatient study. Respiration 2009;78(3):293–300.

41. Mahajan A, Patel S, Hogarth D, et al. Electromagnetic navigational bronchoscopy: an effective and safe approach to diagnose peripheral lung lesions unreachable by conventional bronchoscopy in high-risk patients. J Bronchology Interv Pulmonol 2011;18(2):133–7.

42. Pearlstein DP, Quinn CC, Burtis CC, et al. Electromagnetic navigation bronchoscopy performed by thoracic surgeons: one center's early success. Ann Thorac Surg 2012;93(3):944–9 [discussion: 949–50].

43. Loo F, Halligan A, Port J, et al. The emerging technique of electromagnetic navigation bronchoscopy-guided fine-needle aspiration of peripheral lung lesions: promising results in 50 lesions. Cancer Cytopathol 2014;122(3):191–9.

From Diagnosis to Treatment
Clinical Applications of Nanotechnology in Thoracic Surgery

Christopher S. Digesu, MD[a], Sophie C. Hofferberth, MBBS[a],
Mark W. Grinstaff, PhD[b,c,d],
Yolonda L. Colson, MD, PhD[a,e,*]

KEYWORDS

- Nanotechnology • Nanotheranostics • Lung cancer • Thoracic surgery

KEY POINTS

- Nanotechnology is an exciting field of medicine that is rapidly evolving from in vitro and in vivo testing to the clinical arena.
- Through targeted drug delivery, nanoparticles (NPs) are able to deliver therapeutics at increased local concentrations with minimal systemic toxicity.
- A variety of material platforms are currently available with specific advantages and disadvantages.
- With more research into the mechanisms of action and safety profiles, NPs promise to be a major part of medicine and surgery moving forward.
- Thoracic surgery may benefit from improved diagnostic imaging, advancements in image-guided surgery, and the enhanced efficacy profile of targeted and stimuli-responsive drug delivery.

INTRODUCTION

Nanotechnology is a rapidly evolving field that offers novel opportunities for the treatment and diagnosis of oncologic disease, specifically in thoracic surgery. The use of nanoparticles (NPs), materials generally ranging in size from 1 to 1000 nm, has emerged from the desire to achieve targeted drug delivery that maximizes treatment efficacy, while minimizing toxicity.[1-3] To achieve

This work was supported with funding from the National Science Foundation (DMR-1006601) and the National Institutes of Health (R01CA131044, R01CA149561, R25 CA153955, T32 CA009535).
The authors have no disclosures.
This work was supported in part by Brigham and Women's Hospital Center for Surgical Innovation, Boston University Center for Integration of Medicine and Innovative Technology, Boston University Nanomedicine Program and Cross-Disciplinary Training in Nanotechnology for Cancer, and Brigham and Women's Hospital Advanced Training in Surgical Oncology.
^a Division of Thoracic Surgery, Department of Surgery, Brigham and Women's Hospital, 15 Francis St, Boston, MA 02115, USA; ^b Department of Biomedical Engineering, Metcalf Science Center, Boston University, SCI 518, 590 Commonwealth Avenue, Boston, MA 02215, USA; ^c Department of Chemistry, Metcalf Science Center, Boston University, SCI 518, 590 Commonwealth Avenue, Boston, MA 02215, USA; ^d Department of Medicine, Metcalf Science Center, Boston University, SCI 518, 590 Commonwealth Avenue, Boston, MA 02215, USA; ^e Division of Thoracic Surgery, Brigham and Women's Hospital, Harvard Medical School, 15 Francis St, Boston, MA 02155, USA
* Corresponding author. Division of Thoracic Surgery, Brigham and Women's Hospital, Harvard Medical School, 15 Francis St, Boston, MA 02155.
E-mail address: ycolson@partners.org

Thorac Surg Clin 26 (2016) 215–228
http://dx.doi.org/10.1016/j.thorsurg.2015.12.009
1547-4127/16/$ – see front matter © 2016 Elsevier Inc. All rights reserved.

this goal, NPs are being engineered with varying characteristics and increasing complexity. Researchers leverage the chemical and physical characteristics of small molecule drugs, peptides, proteins, nucleic acids, lipids, polymers, and elemental metals to form a number of unique NPs. These NPs can be enhanced further through a variety of approaches, such as surface modification and responsiveness to the tumor microenvironment, leading to improved pharmacology and active intracellular function.[4]

Nanotechnology has broad application in the field of oncology; however, thoracic oncology is uniquely poised to benefit given the relatively poor prognosis of thoracic malignancies, such as lung and esophageal cancers, as well as the intricacy of the thoracic cavity, which requires careful navigation. Lung cancer is among the most common malignancies and is the number one cause of cancer-related death in the United States.[5] With recent guidelines for lung cancer screening from the National Lung Screening Trial, it is anticipated that the incidence of lung cancer will increase dramatically, and thus the number of patients requiring treatment.[6] Nanotechnology will change the way we approach lung cancer in the future, both as an adjunct to thoracic surgery by improving preoperative diagnosis, intraoperative tumor localization, and image-guided lymphatic mapping, as well as to thoracic oncology through improved systemic therapy of more advanced disease. For example, traditional chemotherapeutics such as paclitaxel and doxorubicin, which are typically used to treat lung cancer, are being packaged within the various nanotechnologies to enhance the pharmacokinetics and biodistribution of drug resulting in improved local concentration. Traditional contrast agents used for computed tomography (CT) and MRI are being delivered via novel nanostructures to provide improved imaging and diagnostic capabilities, and fluorescent nanomarkers are guiding surgeons to the exact tumor location and associated lymphatics.[7–9] Clearly, nanotechnology has the potential to impact each stage from the diagnosis to the treatment of thoracic malignancy as researchers are able to tailor composition, structure, and properties to meet the challenges of clinical application.

MATERIAL PLATFORMS FOR NANOTECHNOLOGY

Nanotechnology comprises a variety of platforms, including nanocrystals, polymeric NPs, liposomes, quantum dots, micelles, dendrimers, and carbon nanotubes (CNTs; **Fig. 1**). Each platform possesses distinctive properties such as size, shape, charge, and surface characteristics that can be strategically altered to overcome the physiologic challenges faced by traditional chemotherapeutics. Commonly used antineoplastic agents in lung cancer, such as paclitaxel or docetaxel, are often difficult to solubilize with nonspecific targeting leading to a vast array of unwanted side effects; however, encapsulation of drugs in NPs facilitates improved biocompatibility and biodistribution, protects against acidic or enzymatic breakdown, and importantly allows for targeted delivery of drug to tumor-laden tissue.[10–12] Tumor neovascularization leads to increased permeability allowing NPs to passively accumulate and remain within tumor tissue through the enhanced permeability and retention effect, a key mechanism driving NP-mediated tumor targeting (**Fig. 2**).[4] In addition, NPs can be engineered with a variety of targeting moieties (ie, ligands, aptamers, or antibodies) that allow active targeting of specific tumors.[13] NPs are modified to provide diagnostic and therapeutic capabilities tailored to specific clinical applications through drug or gene loading, endogenous or exogenous stimuli, contrast or dye loading, or even a combination of these. The distinct advantages and disadvantages of common material platforms are outlined elsewhere in this paper, with a focus on specific innovations that are certain to impact the field of thoracic oncology.

Nanocrystals

Nanocrystals are pure drugs that have been processed down to nanometer size, typically 100 to 1000 nm. Drug processing is achieved using a variety of methods including 'bottom-up' (precipitation) or 'top-down' (high-pressure homogenization) approaches.[14,15] The advantages of nanocrystal drug delivery stem from high saturation solubility owing to a small size and an amorphous state.[16] Nanocrystals can be altered using surface modifiers such as polyethylene glycol to avoid opsonization and consumption by the reticuloendothelial system, allowing for passive tumor accumulation via the enhanced permeability and retention effect.[14] Traditional chemotherapeutics such as paclitaxel are being processed into nanocrystal formulations to take advantage of these properties. For example, paclitaxel is traditionally delivered using a Cremophor EL (polyethoxylated castor oil and ethanol mixture) carrier that is responsible for many of the clinical side effects associated with paclitaxel.[17] Promisingly, paclitaxel-loaded nanocrystals demonstrate significantly less toxicity in preclinical studies using

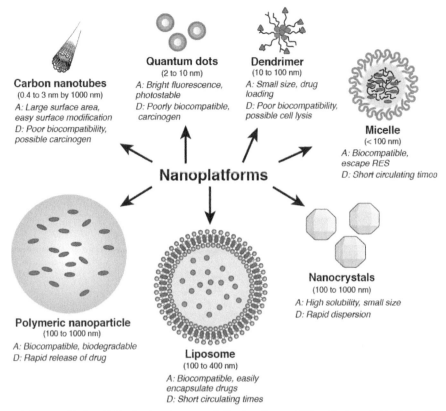

Fig. 1. Nanoplatforms display distinct advantages and disadvantages. RES, reticuloendothelial system.

murine lung cancer models.[18] Nevertheless, further testing is required to better understand the mechanisms of nanocrystal drug delivery as studies show that nanocrystals can rapidly disperse after intravenous administration owing to their high intrinsic solubility, dissolution rate, and rapid dilution.[14]

Quantum Dots

Nanocrystal fluorophores, known as quantum dots, are inorganic fluorescent platforms composed of a heavy metal within a semiconductor shell, ranging from 2 to 10 nm with emissions ranging from 450 to 850 nm based on the size of the quantum dot. Quantum dots exhibit strong light absorbance, bright fluorescence, and marked photostability facilitating their application as a powerful imaging tool. Preclinical studies have successfully used quantum dot technology to visualize tumors and associated lymph nodes after intravenous injection.[19,20] Poor baseline biocompatibility, however, necessitates modification to a hydrophilic state or encapsulation with phospholipids, micelles, polymer beads, and so on, which also permits subsequent attachment of targeting moieties.[21] Despite significant interest, clinical translation of quantum dots has been slow owing to concerns over heavy metal toxicity. Heavy metals such as cadmium, frequently used in quantum dots, can be toxic, particularly if released after exposure to unstable surface coating.[22] Although clinical applicability does remain a possibility; as recent studies by Lin and colleagues[23] showed in a long-term murine model no observable toxicity in mice exposed to novel non–cadmium-based quantum dots.

Liposomes

Liposomes, one of the first described nanosized drug delivery systems, are spherical, bilayer platforms composed of amphiphilic phospholipids (and cholesterol) ranging in size from 100 to 400 nm.[1,2,24] They are ideal in their ability to encapsulate traditional chemotherapeutics and/ or other NPs such as quantum dots to form nano-theranostic vehicles. In addition, they are biocompatible with low toxicity and immunogenicity.[25] Initially, short circulating times owing to opsonization inhibited clinical applicability, however, PEGylation led to longer circulating times and the eventual approval by the US Food and Drug Administration of liposomal doxorubicin, known

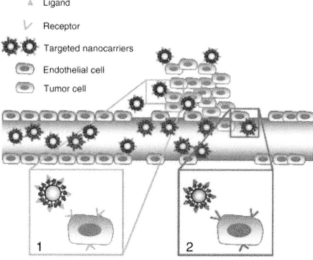

Fig. 2. Tumor targeting of nanoparticles. (*A*) Permeable vasculature from endothelial cell gaps leads to passive diffusion of small molecules and nanocarriers into the tumor microenvironment. Owing to their size, nanocarriers do not diffuse out as easily and hence accumulate within the tumor tissue. (*B*) Specific receptors on nanocarriers target ligands on the tumor tissue. (*From* Danhier F, Oliver F, Veronique P. To exploit the tumor microenvironment: Passive and active tumor targeting of nanocarriers for anti-cancer drug delivery. J Control Release 2010;148(2):5; with permission from Elsevier.)

as Doxil.[2] Multiple studies report the liposomal formulation of other traditional chemotherapeutics such as paclitaxel for treatment of lung cancer via intravenous and inhalational therapies.[26,27]

Dendrimers

Dendrimers are highly branched, synthetic, nano-size (10–100 nm) molecules created from the repetitive addition of branching units to an amine core. Drugs can be encapsulated to improve solubility or attached to the surface for delivery.[28] Newer generations of dendrimers are more hydrophobic, exhibit improved drug stability, and allow specific targeting through increasingly complex branching.[24] For example, Majoros and colleagues[29] demonstrated enhanced tumor targeting and improved cytotoxicity by conjugating paclitaxel to a poly(amidoamine) dendrimer. In

addition to drug delivery, dendrimers have been conjugated to iron oxide particles and used in combination with MRI to deliver magnetic hyperthermia and subsequent cytotoxicity, whereas dendrimer-entrapped gold particles have been used to enhance CT imaging of human lung adenocarcinoma.[30,31] Similar to other platforms, cationic dendrimers are subject to unwanted toxicities owing to interaction with cellular membranes that can lead to destabilization and potential cell lysis.[32,33] In addition, Jones and colleagues[34] demonstrated that certain dendrimers with cationic charge can result in platelet aggregation and alpha granule secretion.

Carbon Nanotubes

CNTs are graphene sheets rolled into cylinders measuring 0.4 to 3 nm in diameter and up to

1000 nm in length. Cylinders can be single or rolled concentrically to form single-walled, double-walled, or multiwalled CNTs.[35] CNTs are hydrophobic and thus generally not soluble in aqueous solutions. To improve biocompatibility, surface functionalization must occur, which also presents an opportunity for ligand binding for tumor-specific targeting. In vitro studies using CNTs, show a dose-dependent tumor suppression of human breast cancer cells, and more recently the use of short intervening RNA (siRNA) vectors has demonstrated the eradication of lung cancer xenografts. Although promising, CNTs have led to systemic toxicity in multiple studies. Large surface area, hydrophobicity, insolubility, and a tendency to aggregate, in addition to a serious concern for possible carcinogenesis are all factors that limit the clinical translational of CNTs to date.[36,37] In a study by Kanno and colleagues[38] multiwalled CNTs induced mesothelioma when given to p53 heterozygous mice. Carcinogenesis has been also reported in other studies, and it is postulated that the mechanism is similar to that of asbestos.[35]

Polymeric Nanoparticles

Polymeric NPs are manufactured using a variety of materials and techniques resulting in biocompatible and biodegradable polymers that can be either natural or synthetic, generally ranging from 100 to 1000 nm. Poly(lactic acid) and poly(lactic-co-glycolic acid) polymers are the most widely used synthetic polymers, because their lactic acid and glycolic acid monomers can be easily hydrolyzed and eliminated.[24,39] Natural polymers such as chitosan or dextran have also been used in polymeric NP production. Polymeric NPs offer unique advantages for drug delivery given their particularly capacity to encapsulate and protect drugs from degradation as well as the ability to introduce specific functionality via surface modification.[40] Polymeric-drug conjugated with surface modification, such as doxorubicin-loaded poly(lactic-co-glycolic acid)-polyethylene glycol NPs with conjugated peptide specific for EGFR, demonstrate improved cytotoxicity in vitro (a 62.4 reduction in the median inhibition concentration when compared with free doxorubicin) as well as in vivo tumor accumulation.[41] In addition, clinical trials investigating polymer-conjugated doxorubicin have shown improved antitumor cytotoxicity and decreased systemic toxicity compared with drug alone.[42] More recently, a phase III clinical trial comparing polyglutamic acid conjugated paclitaxel in patients with non–small-cell lung cancer revealed significantly fewer severe side effects compared with traditional chemotherapies.[43,44]

Although promising, polymeric NPs, specifically poly(lactic acid) and poly(lactic-co-glycolic acid), are limited by relatively rapid "burst" release of encapsulated drug, regardless of whether it is in the tumor. Short duration of random drug release has been a driving force behind more targeted structures as well as an interest in environment-responsive polymeric NPs.[40]

Micelles

Micelles are colloidal structures, typically less than 100 nm, with a hydrophobic core and a hydrophilic shell that allows for transport of poorly water soluble agents.[24,45] Clinical trials have been conducted on a micellar formulation containing paclitaxel known as Genexol-PM. In a multicenter phase II trial, Genexol-PM was administered intravenously with cisplatin to patients with advanced non–small-cell lung cancer demonstrating a significant improved median survival time and minimal associated toxicity.[46] Micelles offer a distinct advantage in providing an oral route for some drugs, avoiding renal exclusion, and escaping the reticuloendothelial system. Most toxicity, however, comes from premature release of encapsulated drug.[47]

POTENTIAL CLINICAL APPLICATION OF NANOTECHNOLOGY IN THORACIC SURGERY

Nanotechnology has the potential to advance the field of thoracic surgery by improving the diagnosis, staging, treatment, and therapeutic monitoring of intrathoracic malignancies (**Fig. 3**). Through optimization of the material platforms to overcome their limitations, scientists are discovering how to meet the clinical needs of patients. The sensitivity and specificity of imaging is being improved through nanocarrier contrast agents. Surgeons can more accurately localize a lesion intraoperatively while carefully examining the associated lymphatics. Drugs as well as inhibitory genetic material are being delivered in a "smart" fashion through stimuli-responsive platforms. All of these advancements have led to the emergence of "nanotheranostic" multifunctional NPs to meet the challenges of clinical applicability. Some of the exciting new applications are highlighted.

Nanotechnology in Imaging: Diagnostics and Intraoperative Platforms

NPs engineered as an adjunct to imaging modalities are evolving rapidly to meet the needs of cancer diagnosis. Specifically, contrast agents are being loaded on the surface or encapsulated within NPs to improve imaging sensitivity and

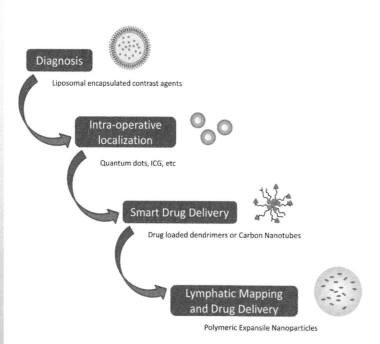

Fig. 3. Nanoparticles participate in each step from diagnosis of cancer to the various forms of treatment. Nanoparticles can be engineered to function at multiple different steps and in combination with each other. ICG, indocyanine green.

specificity while minimizing systemic toxicity. Contrast agents such as supermagnetic iron oxide NPs that are tagged with tumor-specific antibodies (ie, vascular endothelial growth factor) for direct tumor targeting are improving MRI resolution and tumor identification.[48–50] Traditional contrast agents formulated onto nanocarriers better facilitate intratumoral uptake and minimize nephrotoxicity, as demonstrated by gadolinium NPs for MRI and liposomal iodinated contrast agents for CT.[51,52] These improvements have the potential to greatly improve lung cancer diagnosis and staging, particularly given the suboptimal diagnostic accuracy (79%) and sensitivity (64%) of conventional CT-PET scans as well as the risk for nephrotoxicity associated with each intravenous dose of traditional iodinated contrast.[53]

Nanotechnology is also a useful tool in identifying and targeting tumors intraoperatively, particularly given the complex and intricate anatomy of the thoracic cavity. With the new lung cancer screening guidelines, an increasing incidence of early stage cancers presents thoracic surgeons with the challenge of finding smaller, nonpalpable tumors during surgery.[54] Therefore, a strong need for image-guided surgery exists to enable precise tumor resection with maximal parenchymal sparing and avoidance of critical structures. Using murine and rabbit models, 1 group formulated liposomal encapsulated iodohexal, an iodinated contrast agent, and indocyanine green (ICG), a near-infrared fluorescent dye, for dual preoperative and intraoperative tumor localization. Rabbits were inoculated with rabbit lung cancer, VX2, and given the novel liposomal formulation. At 4 days after injection tumor deposits correlated with preoperative CT images and with intraoperative near infrared (NIR) signals.[55,56]

A particular area of thoracic surgery to significantly benefit from the field of nanotechnology is that of lymphatic mapping. Lymph node involvement in non–small-cell lung cancer plays an important role in the staging and overall prognosis of patients with lung cancer. For those patients that are clinically node negative, approximately 30% of clinical stage 1, patients will be upstaged after surgery.[57] Given the poor prognosis associated with nodal involvement and the variable location, extensive lymphadenectomy has become the standard of care; however, it is not without morbidity. This has prompted an exploration into sentinel lymph node (SLN) mapping whereby tumor draining lymph nodes can undergo more in-depth immunohistochemical analysis. Early human clinical trials used methylene blue and [99]technetium, although neither are ideal for thoracic surgery.[58,59] More recently, NIR technology, which detects light emitted in the 700 to 900 nm range, and ICG, which migrates from the tumor to the SLN, have been used in combination to improve mapping and biopsy of SLN. In a clinical trial, patients with non–small cell lung cancer underwent peritumoral ICG injection. Here 26 NIR plus SLNs were identified in 15 patients, with 7 NIR plus SLNs (from 6 patients) harboring metastatic disease on histologic analysis, which demonstrated 100% SLN identification and 100% correlation of SLN pathology with overall nodal status in lung cancer.[60] Another study leveraged the fluorescent capabilities of quantum dots with direct injection into the lung parenchyma. In this porcine model, a bright fluorescent signal could be visualized in real time migrating to the SLN within minutes.[61] Similar results were noted for lymphatic mapping of the pleural space and esophagus.[62,63]

Stimuli-Responsive Drug Release Nanoparticles

A major area of nanotechnology application is in smart drug delivery and cancer therapeutics. Paclitaxel, a taxane that stabilizes microtubules and exhibits cytotoxicity against numerous solid tumors, and doxorubicin, an anthracycline that intercalates a host cell's DNA, are 2 common chemotherapeutic agents employed.[17,64] Numerous studies have demonstrated superior in vitro and in vivo tumor cytotoxicity when these agents are incorporated into a NP.[27,29,65,66] For example, using a murine xenograft model a paclitaxel chitosan based micellar formulation displayed significant tumor reduction (P <.01) and less morbidity (approximated by body weight loss) compared with intravenous paclitaxel.[67] These studies represent the improved delivery of chemotherapeutic drug to tumor. In addition, other studies have shown that NPs can function synergistically with known chemotherapies.

The ultimate goal of NP drug delivery is to achieve targeted and controlled drug release within the tumor. Pursuit of this goal has led to engineering of stimuli-responsive NPs that can be triggered either to act or to release a therapeutic agent based on a specific endogenous microenvironment or an external stimulus. Examples of endogenous and exogenous stimuli being exploited include light, pH or temperature change, applied magnetism, redox environment, or

enzymes (**Fig. 4**).[40,68] Numerous studies are being devised to leverage stimuli unique to cancer cells or other pathologic states, making it clear that the next generation of nanoplatforms will have a "responsive " functionality to aid in the targeted release of a drug payload as a function of a biologic event or microenvironment.

Many polymeric NPs are limited in their clinical translation owing to the relatively rapid release of encapsulated drug. As such, stimuli-responsive polymers have been engineered to allow for delayed, tumor-targeted release of drug in response to a tumor microenvironment. For example, acidic pH within the tumor microenvironment or endosome is well-characterized and has been used as a "trigger" for chemotherapy release at the site of intracavitary tumors such as mesothelioma.[40] Upon encountering an environmental of pH 5 or less, as occurs in endosomes, cleavage of a protecting group changes the NP polymer from hydrophobic to hydrophilic with significant expansion of NP size and resultant drug release (**Fig. 5**). The intracellular targeting of chemotherapy release as a function of pH has resulted in markedly superior tumor cytotoxicity and improved survival in in vivo studies.[69,70]

Similarly, redox-sensitive NPs have emerged as another popular approach to responsively trigger drug release.[71] Glutathione levels are 2 to 3 times greater within the cytosol of animal cells and undergo a reduction-oxidative reaction with glutathione disulfide, leading to the release of drug. Loaded drug can be further released via redox reaction within the lysosome. NPs encapsulating doxorubicin were prepared with disulfide bonds to allow for triggered intracellular drug release. Subsequent in vivo fluorescent imaging revealed tumor specific targeting and drug release as can be seen in **Fig. 6**.[72]

In contrast, photodynamic therapy has been used as an exogenous stimulus to "activate" nanostructures against a variety of malignancies. Using a combination of a photosensitizer and a light

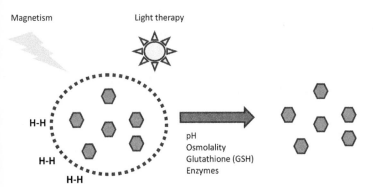

Magnetism   Light therapy

H-H

H-H

H-H

pH
Osmolality
Glutathione (GSH)
Enzymes

Fig. 4. Stimuli-responsive nanoparticles. A variety of endogenous and exogenous stimuli can induce a specific action or release of drug.

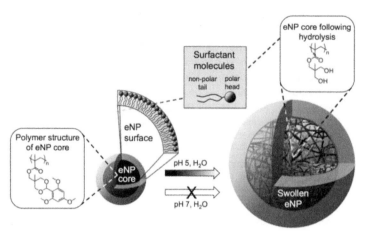

Fig. 5. The pH responsive expansile nanoparticles (eNP) expand to release drug when in the presence of a pH of 5. (*Adapted from* Stolzoff M, Ekladious I, Colby AH, et al. Synthesis and characterization of hybrid polymer/lipid expansile nanoparticles: imparting surface functionality for targeting and stability. Biomacromolecules. 2015;16(7):14; with permission from American Chemical Society, Copyright (2015).)

source, free radical oxygen species can be generated to induce cell death via localized hyperthermia, apoptosis, or induction of an immune response.[73] Photosensitizers such as porfimer sodium and ICG have been packaged within nanostructures (ie, porfimer sodium-liposomal system) to limit systemic exposure and decrease side effects such as generalized photosensitivity, but permit for direct photodynamic or photothermal cell cytotoxicity.[74,75] Other studies have

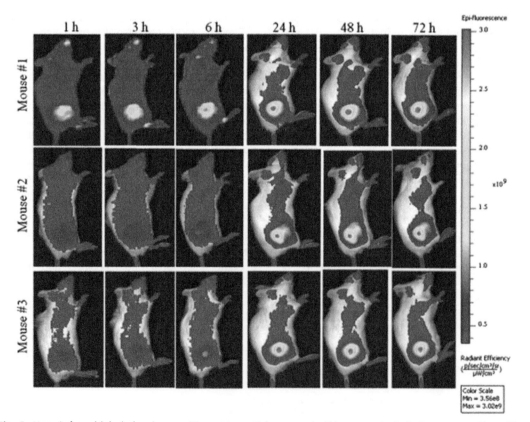

Fig. 6. Near infrared-labeled redox-sensitive nanoparticles reproducibly concentrate in tumor over time. (*From* Nguyen CT, Tran TH, Amiji M, et al. Redox-sensitive nanoparticles from amphiphilic cholesterol-based block copolymers for enhanced tumor intracellular release of doxorubicin. Nanomedicine. 2015;11(8):14; with permission from Elsevier.)

similarly examined the use of applied near-infrared light to induce the release of drug into the local environment.[76]

Lymphatic Drug Delivery

New research has focused on the delivery of chemotherapy specifically to the lymphatics and the treatment of occult lymph node metastases. This work has led to studies investigating chemotherapy drug concentrations within the tumor and the draining lymph nodes as a function of the method of drug delivery. Interestingly, drug levels are as much 180 to 300 times lower in both tumor and lymph nodes after intravenous administration as opposed to peritumoral injection.[77] As a result, local peritumoral NP delivery is being explored as a unique approach to increase substantially the level of chemotherapeutic agent within both the tumor and lymph nodes. Exploiting the stimuli-dependent release of drug seen in expansile NPs, a murine xenograft model of triple negative breast cancer cells with a propensity for lymph node metastasis was used to assess the ability of paclitaxel loaded expansile NP (pax-eNP) to control disease. The pax-eNP accumulated in the lymph nodes and were present even after 10 days, a stark contrast to systemic paclitaxel, which has a half-life of only 7 hours. There was also a significant decrease in the percentage of lymph node metastasis present 6.5 weeks after peritumoral pax-eNP therapy (33% nodal metastasis with pax-eNP and 100% nodal metastasis with unloaded eNP and only; $P <.005$).[70] Prevention of nodal metastasis using nanotechnology to target and enhance drug delivery has the potential to have a major impact on early stage cancers after operative resection.

Active Tumor-Targeting Platforms

Other investigators have focused on mechanisms for directing nanostructures to a target tumor with enhanced specificity. Epidermal growth factor receptor (EGFR) is expressed in approximately 50% to 80% of non–small cell lung cancers and typically has a poor prognosis, making it an ideal therapeutic target. NPs conjugated to cetuximab, a monoclonal antibody to EGFR, have been tested in a murine model of EGFR-positive non–small cell lung cancer. Tumor volume was significantly less and there was no overall weight loss in the cetuximab-NP group when compared with cetuximab alone. Tumor migration and EGFR intracellular signaling were also decreased.[78] Further investigation into the mechanism of cetuximab conjugated plasmonic magnetic NPs revealed induced autophagy, which was not seen in cetuximab alone indicating an added degree of cytotoxicity when conjugated to a nanoparticle.[79]

Nanoparticles for Gene Delivery

The siRNA segments can target specific mRNA sequences and affect gene translation via the RNA-induced silencing complex, as in **Fig. 7**.[80,81] However, clinical translation has been elusive owing to poor cellular uptake of nucleic acids, the lack of biocompatible siRNA carriers, rapid degradation by nucleases, and accelerated renal excretion.[82] In an in vivo murine xenograft model of human lung adenocarcinoma, Chen and colleagues[83] used a novel system of magnetic mesoporous silica NPs loaded with vascular endothelial growth factor siRNA, capped with polyethylenimine, and PEGylated for biocompatibility. Mice subjected to the siRNA NP showed marked tumor suppression, decreased tumor metastasis, and overall improved survival while maintaining favorable tissue biocompatibility and biosafety. In another study, multiwalled CNTs were loaded with siRNA specific for PLK1. Intratumoral injection of human lung cancer xenografts led to drastically reduced tumor growth and increased survival.[84] A major target in siRNA delivery for lung cancer is the KRAS protooncogene, one of the most common oncogenes in human cancers that typically portends a poor prognosis. Using a nanoliposomal delivery system for KRAS siRNA, 1 group found a 90% reduction in KRAS on Western blot analysis, significant tumor reduction (50% vs 6% in negative control siRNA), and reduced distant metastasis. Numerous other studies are looking at a variety of targets for siRNA (ie, tissue factor, HDM2, AKT1) incorporated onto an array of basic NP platforms with increasing levels of sophistication.[82]

NANOTHERANOSTICS: A NEW FRONTIER IN THORACIC SURGERY

With increasing knowledge of NPs and their capabilities, a new field known as nanotheranostics has evolved in an effort to deliver diagnostic and therapeutic properties on a single, unified platform. For example, multiple nanotechnologies can be combined to take advantage of their distinctive properties. Typical nanotheranostic agents may include a polymer component for stabilization and biocompatibility, an encapsulated therapeutic agent such as a traditional chemotherapeutic drug or siRNA, and an imaging agent such as a fluorophore or contrast agent (**Fig. 8**). Researchers recently encapsulated the MRI contrast agent supermagnetic iron oxide with doxorubicin using the copolymer maleimide-polythylene

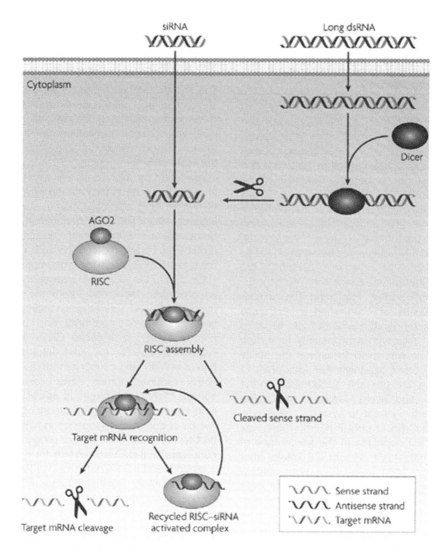

Fig. 7. Short intervening RNA (siRNA) can be introduced via nanocarrier or double-stranded DNA that is cleaved by the Dicer enzyme within the cell. The siRNA is then incorporated into the RNA-induced silencing complex (RISC) leading to cleavage of target messenger RNA (mRNA) and thus silencing of the targeted gene. dsRNA, double-stranded RNA. (*Reprinted from* Whitehead KA, Langer R, Anderson DR. Knocking down barriers: advances in siRNA delivery. Nat Rev Drug Dis 2009;8(2):16; with permission from Macmillan Publishers Ltd, copyright (2009).)

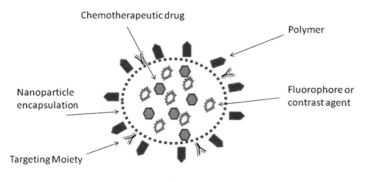

Fig. 8. Nanotheranositics. These agents combine many properties of the basic nanoparticles to form single platforms capable of both diagnostics and therapeutics.

glycol-poly(lactic acid) to allow for preoperative imaging with MRI while delivering chemotherapy all on a single, biocompatible platform.[85] In another study, quantum dots and supermagnetic iron oxide were coupled on a chitosan-based NP platform with folate conjugates for tumor targeting and then loaded with chemotherapeutic camptothecin.[86]

Nanotheranostics are particularly useful in providing surgeons with the opportunity to perform an ideal resection while delivering therapy at the same time. Given the known potential for toxicity associated with quantum dots, some studies have explored the use of small pH-responsive NPs labeled with an NIR fluorophore that also carries paclitaxel to the SLN. Evaluation of this technology in a large animal model demonstrated rapid detection of the SLN upon operative exploration and significant concentration of both the fluorophore and paclitaxel.[87,88] As toxicities of current NPs being engineered to encapsulate both fluorophore and chemotherapeutic drug continue to be delineated, newer nanotheranositic systems have the potential to maximize the benefit of surgery.

Treatment of lung cancer will benefit strongly from the emerging field of nanotheranostics given the poor response to traditional chemotherapies, overall poor prognosis, and difficult surgical anatomy associated with the thoracic cavity. As more early stage lung cancers are discovered, we are at an ideal time to employ nanotheranostics by simultaneously aiding surgeons in finding non-palpable nodules, biopsying sentinel nodes instead of the traditional lymphadenectomy, and delivering chemotherapy to the targeted tumor.

SUMMARY

Nanotechnology is an exciting field of medicine that is evolving rapidly from in vitro and in vivo testing to the clinical arena. Through targeted drug delivery, NPs are able to deliver therapeutics at increased local concentrations with minimal systemic toxicity. A variety of material platforms are available currently with specific advantages and disadvantages. With more research into the mechanisms of action and safety profiles, NPs promise to be a major part of medicine and surgery moving forward. Thoracic surgery stands to benefit from the improved diagnostic imaging, advancements in image-guided surgery through tumor localization and lymphatic mapping, and from the enhanced efficacy profile of targeted and stimuli-responsive drug delivery. Most promising is the creation of nanotheranostic systems that integrate each of these advances into a single,

unified platform. This new frontier in oncologic therapy promises to transform the care of thoracic surgery patients moving forward.

REFERENCES

1. Farokhzad OC, Langer R. Impact of nanotechnology on drug delivery. ACS Nano 2009;3(1):16–20.
2. Heath JR, Davis ME. Nanotechnology and cancer. Annu Rev Med 2008;59:2251–65.
3. Ferrari M. Cancer nanotechnology: opportunities and challenges. Nat Rev Cancer 2005, 5(3):161–71.
4. Zhu L, Torchilin VP. Stimulus-responsive nanopreparations for tumor targeting. Integr Biol (Camb) 2013; 5(1):96–107.
5. Howlader N, Noone AM, Krapcho M, et al, editors. SEER cancer statistics review, 1975-2012. Bethesda (MD): National Cancer Institute. Available at: http://seer.cancer.gov/csr/1975_2012/. Accessed August 10, 2015.
6. Yanagawa J, Rusch VW. Current surgical therapy for stage IIIA (N2) non-small cell lung cancer. Semin Thorac Cardiovasc Surg 2011;23(4):291–6.
7. Ma P, Mumper RJ. Paclitaxel nano-delivery systems: a comprehensive review. J Nanomed Nanotechnol 2013;4(2):1000164.
8. Badea CT, Athreya KK, Espinosa G, et al. Computed tomography imaging of primary lung cancer in mice using a liposomal-iodinated contrast agent. PLoS One 2012;7(4):e34496.
9. Hill TK, Abdulahad A, Kelkar SS, et al. Indocyanine green-loaded nanoparticles for image-guided tumor surgery. Bioconjug Chem 2015;26(2):294–303.
10. Sahoo SK, Labhasetwar V. Nanotech approaches to drug delivery and imaging. Drug Discov Today 2003;8(24):1112–20.
11. Zhang G, Zeng X, Li P. Nanomaterials in cancer-therapy drug delivery system. J Biomed Nanotechnol 2013;9(5):741–50.
12. Biswas S, Deshpande PP, Perche F, et al. Octa-arginine-modified pegylated liposomal doxorubicin: an effective treatment strategy for non-small cell lung cancer. Cancer Lett 2013;335(1):191–200.
13. Bazak R, Houri M, El Achy S, et al. Cancer active targeting by nanoparticles: a comprehensive review of literature. J Cancer Res Clin Oncol 2015;141(5): 769–84.
14. Gao L, Liu G, Ma J, et al. Drug nanocrystals: in vivo performances. J Control Release 2012;160(3):418–30.
15. Pawar VK, Singh Y, Meher JG, et al. Engineered nanocrystal technology: in-vivo fate, targeting and applications in drug delivery. J Control Release 2014;183:51–66.
16. Junghanns JU, Müller RH. Nanocrystal technology, drug delivery and clinical applications. Int J Nanomedicine 2008;3(3):295–309.

17. Joshi M, Liu X, Belani CP. Taxanes, past, present, and future impact on non-small cell lung cancer. Anticancer Drugs 2014;25(5):571–83.

18. Liu F, Park JY, Zhang Y, et al. Targeted cancer therapy with novel high drug-loading nanocrystals. J Pharm Sci 2010;99(8):3542–51.

19. Azzazy HM, Mansour MM, Kazmierczak SC. From diagnostics to therapy: prospects of quantum dots. Clin Biochem 2007;40(13–14):917–27.

20. Schulz MD, Khullar O, Frangioni JV, et al. Nanotechnology in thoracic surgery. Ann Thorac Surg 2010; 89(6):S2188–90.

21. Akerman ME, Chan WC, Laakkonen P, et al. Nanocrystal targeting in vivo. Proc Natl Acad Sci U S A 2002;99(20):12617–21.

22. Bottrill M, Green M. Some aspects of quantum dot toxicity. Chem Commun (Camb) 2011;47(25): 7039–50.

23. Lin G, Ouyang Q, Hu R, et al. In vivo toxicity assessment of non-cadmium quantum dots in BALB/c mice. Nanomedicine 2015;11(2):341–50.

24. Muthu MS, Leong DT, Mei L, et al. Nanotheranostics - application and further development of nanomedicine strategies for advanced theranostics. Theranostics 2014;4(6):660–77.

25. Kraft JC, Freeling JP, Wang Z, et al. Emerging Research and clinical development trends of liposome and lipid nanoparticle drug delivery systems. J Pharm Sci 2014;103(1):29–52.

26. Wang X, Zhou J, Wang Y, et al. A phase I clinical and pharmacokinetic study of paclitaxel liposome infused in non-small cell lung cancer patients with malignant pleural effusions. Eur J Cancer 2010; 46(8):1474–80.

27. Guo Y, Wang L, Lv P, et al. Transferrin-conjugated doxorubicin-loaded lipid-coated nanoparticles for the targeting and therapy of lung cancer. Oncol Lett 2015;9(3):1065–72.

28. Steichen SD, Caldorera-Moore M, Peppas NA. A review of current nanoparticle and targeting moieties for the delivery of cancer therapeutics. Eur J Pharm Sci 2013;48(3):416–27.

29. Majoros IJ, Myc A, Thomas T, et al. PAMAM dendrimer-based multifunctional conjugate for cancer therapy: synthesis, characterization, and functionality. Biomacromolecules 2006;7(2):572–9.

30. Walter A, Billotey C, Garofalo A, et al. Mastering the shape and composition of dendronized iron oxide nanoparticles to tailor magnetic resonance imaging and hyperthermia. Chem Mater 2014; 26(18):5252–64.

31. Wang H, Zheng L, Peng C, et al. Folic acid-modified dendrimer-entrapped gold nanoparticles as nanoprobes for targeted CT imaging of human lung adenocarcinoma. Biomaterials 2013;34(2): 470–80.

32. Fischer D, Li Y, Ahlemeyer B, et al. In vitro cytotoxicity testing of polycations: influence of polymer structure on cell viability and hemolysis. Biomaterials 2003;24(7):1121–31.

33. Madaan K, Kumar S, Poonia N, et al. Dendrimers in drug delivery and targeting: drug-dendrimer interactions and toxicity issues. J Pharm Bioallied Sci 2014;6(3):139–50.

34. Jones CF, Campbell RA, Franks Z, et al. Cationic PAMAM dendrimers disrupt key platelet functions. Mol Pharmacol 2012;9(6):1599–611.

35. Rastogi V, Yadav P, Bhattacharya SS, et al. Carbon nanotubes: an emerging drug carrier for targeting cancer cells. J Drug Deliv 2014;2014:670815.

36. Rodriguez-Yanez Y, Munoz B, Albores A. Mechanisms of toxicity by carbon nanotubes. Toxicol Mech Methods 2013;23(3):178–95.

37. Takagi A, Hirose A, Nishimura T, et al. Induction of mesothelioma in p53+/- mouse by intraperitoneal application of multi-wall carbon nanotube. J Toxicol Sci 2008;33(1):105–16.

38. Kanno J, Takagi A, Hirose A, et al. Induction of mesothelioma in p53+/- mouse by intraperitoneal application of multi-wall carbon nanotube. J Toxicol Sci 2008;33(1):105–16.

39. Wang AZ, Langer R, Farokhzad OC. Nanoparticle delivery of cancer drugs. Annu Rev Med 2012;63: 185–98.

40. Colson YL, Grinstaff MW. Biologically responsive polymeric nanoparticles for drug delivery. Adv Mater 2012;24(28):3878–86.

41. Liu CW, Lin WJ. Polymeric nanoparticles conjugate a novel heptapeptide as an epidermal growth factor receptor-active targeting ligand for doxorubicin. Int J Nanomedicine 2012;7:4749–67.

42. Vasey PA, Kaye SB, Morrison R, et al. Phase I clinical and pharmacokinetic study of PK1 [N-(2-hydroxypropyl)methacrylamide copolymer doxorubicin]: first member of a new class of chemotherapeutic agents-drug-polymer conjugates. Clin Cancer Res 1999;5(1):83–94.

43. Langer CJ. CT-2103: a novel macromolecular taxane with potential advantages compared with conventional taxanes. Clin Lung Cancer 2004;6(Suppl 2): S85–8.

44. Langer CJ, O'byrne KJ, Socinski MA. Phase III trial comparing paclitaxel poliglumex (CT-2103, PPX) in combination with carboplatin versus standard paclitaxel and carboplatin in the treatment of PS 2 patients with chemotherapy-naive advanced non-small cell lung cancer. J Thorac Oncol 2008;3(6): 623–30.

45. Frank D, Tyagi C, Tomar L, et al. Overview of the role of nanotechnological innovations in the detection and treatment of solid tumors. Int J Nanomedicine 2014;9:589–613.

46. Kim DW, Kim SY, Kim HK, et al. Multicenter phase II trial of Genexol-PM, a novel Cremophor-free, polymeric micelle formulation of paclitaxel, with cisplatin in patients with advanced non-small-cell lung cancer. Ann Oncol 2007;18(12):2009–14.

47. Moghimi SM, Hunter AC, Murray JC, et al. Cellular distribution of nonionic micelles. Science 2004; 303(5658):626–8.

48. Hsieh WJ, Liang CJ, Chieh JJ, et al. In vivo tumor targeting and imaging with anti-vascular endothelial growth factor antibody-conjugated dextran-coated iron oxide nanoparticles. Int J Nanomedicine 2012; 7:2833–42.

49. Mallia RJ, McVeigh PZ, Fisher CJ. Wide-field multiplexed imaging of EGFR- targeted cancers using topical application of NIR SERS nanoprobes. Nanomedicine (Lond) 2015;10(1):89–101.

50. Koyama T, Shimura M, Minemoto Y, et al. Evaluation of selective tumor detection by clinical magnetic resonance imaging using antibody-conjugated superparamagnetic iron oxide. J Control Release 2012;159(3):413–8.

51. Key J, Leary JF. Nanoparticles for multimodal in vivo imaging in nanomedicine. Int J Nanomedicine 2014; 9:711–26.

52. Kong WH, Lee WJ, Cui ZY, et al. Nanoparticulate carrier containing water-insoluble iodinated oil as a multifunctional contrast agent for computed tomography imaging. Biomaterials 2007;28(36): 5555–61.

53. Fischer B, Lassen U, Mortensen J, et al. Preoperative staging of lung cancer with combined PET-CT. N Engl J Med 2009;361(1):32–9.

54. Chen VW, Ruiz BA, Hsieh MC, et al. Analysis of stage and clinical/prognostic factors for lung cancer from SEER registries: AJCC staging and collaborative stage data collection system. Cancer 2014; 120(Suppl 23):3781–92.

55. Zheng J, Muhanna N, De Souza R, et al. A multimodal nano agent for image-guided cancer surgery. Biomaterials 2015;67:160–8.

56. Anayama T, Nakajima T, Dunne M, et al. A novel minimally invasive technique to create a rabbit VX2 lung tumor model for nano-sized image contrast and interventional studies. PLoS One 2013;8(6):e67355.

57. D'Cunha J, Herndon JE, Herzan DL, et al. Poor correspondence between clinical and pathologic staging in stage 1 non-small cell lung cancer: results from CALGB 9761, a prospective trial. Lung Cancer 2005;48(2):241–6.

58. Liptay MJ, D'amico TA, Nwogu C, et al. Intraoperative sentinel node mapping with technitium-99 in lung cancer: results of CALGB 140203 multicenter phase II trial. J Thorac Oncol 2009;4(2):198–202.

59. Rzyman W, Hagen OM, Dziadziuszko R, et al. Blue-dye intraoperative sentinel lymph node mapping in early non-small lung cancer. Eur J Surg Oncol 2006;32(4):462–5.

60. Gilmore DM, Khullar OV, Jaklitsch MT, et al. Identification of metastatic nodal disease in a phase 1 dose-escalation trial of intraoperative sentinel lymph node mapping in non-small cell lung cancer using near-infrared imaging. J Thorac Cardiovasc Surg 2013;146(3):562–70.

61. Soltesz EG, Kim S, Laurence RG, et al. Intraoperative sentinel lymph node mapping of the lung using near-infrared fluorescent quantum dots. Ann Thorac Surg 2005;79(1):269–77.

62. Parungo CP, Colson YL, Kim SW, et al. Sentinel lymph node mapping of the pleural space. Chest 2005;127(5):1799–804.

63. Parungo CP, Ohnishi S, Kim SW, et al. Intraoperative identification of esophageal sentinel lymph nodes with near-infrared fluorescence imaging. J Thorac Cardiovasc Surg 2005;129(4):844–50.

64. Young RC, Ozols RF, Myers CE. The anthracycline antineoplastic drugs. N Engl J Med 1981;305(3): 139–53.

65. Hollis CP, Weiss HL, Evers BM, et al. In vivo investigation of hybrid paclitaxel nanocrystals with dual fluorescent probes for cancer theranostics. Pharm Res 2014;31(6):1450–9.

66. Zhao T, Chen H, Dong Y, et al. Paclitaxel-loaded poly(glycolide-co- ε-caprolactone)-b-D-α-tocopheryl polyethylene glycol 2000 succinate nanoparticles for lung cancer therapy. Int J Nanomedicine 2013;8:1947–57.

67. Zhang C, Qu G, Sun Y, et al. Pharmacokinetics, biodistribution, efficacy and safety of N-octyl-O-sulfate chitosan micelles loaded with paclitaxel. Biomaterials 2008;29(9):1233–41.

68. Cheng R, Meng F, Deng C, et al. Dual and multistimuli responsive polymeric nanoparticles for programmed site-specific drug delivery. Biomaterials 2013;34(14):3647–57.

69. Stolzoff M, Ekladious I, Colby AH, et al. Synthesis and characterization of hybrid polymer/lipid expansile nanoparticles: imparting surface functionality for targeting and stability. Biomacromolecules 2015;16(7):1958–66.

70. Liu R, Gilmore DM, Zubris KA, et al. Prevention of nodal metastases in breast cancer following the lymphatic migration of paclitaxel-loaded expansile nanoparticles. Biomaterials 2013;34(7):1810–9.

71. Cheng R, Feng F, Meng F, et al. Glutathione-responsive nano-vehicles as a promising platform for targeted intracellular drug and gene delivery. J Control Release 2011;152(1):2–12.

72. Nguyen CT, Tran TH, Amiji M, et al. Redox-sensitive nanoparticles from amphiphilic cholesterol-based block copolymers for enhanced tumor intracellular release of doxorubicin. Nanomedicine 2015;11(8): 2071–82.

73. Voon SH, Kiew LV, Lee HB, et al. In vivo studies of nanostructure-based photosensitizers for photodynamic cancer therapy. Small 2014;24:4993–5013.

74. Jiang F, Lilge L, Grenier J, et al. Photodynamic therapy of U87 human glioma in nude rat using liposome-delivered photoforin. Lasers Surg Med 1998;22(2):74–80.

75. Jian WH, Yu TW, Chen CJ, et al. Indocyanine green-encapsulated hybrid polymeric nanomicelles for photothermal cancer therapy. Langmuir 2015; 31(22):6202–10.

76. Yang S, Li N, Liu Z, et al. Amphiphilic copolymer coated upconversion nanoparticles for near-infrared light triggered dual anticancer treatment. Nanoscale 2014;6(24):14903–10.

77. Chen J, Wang L, Yao Q, et al. Drug concentrations in axillary lymph nodes after lymphatic chemotherapy on patients with breast cancer. Breast Cancer Res 2004;6(4):R474–7.

78. Qian Y, Qiu M, Wu Q, et al. Enhanced cytotoxic activity of cetuximab in EGFR-positive lung cancer by conjugating with gold nanoparticles. Sci Rep 2014;4:7490.

79. Kuroda S, Tam J, Roth JA, et al. EGFR-targeted plasmonic magnetic nanoparticles suppress lung tumor growth by abrogating G2/M cell-cycle arrest and inducing DNA damage. Int J Nanomedicine 2014;9:3825–39.

80. Draz MS, Fang BA, Zhang P, et al. Nanoparticle-mediated systemic delivery of siRNA for treatment of cancers and viral infections. Theranostics 2014; 4(9):872–92.

81. Whitehead KA, Langer R, Anderson DG. Knocking down barriers: advances in siRNA delivery. Nat Rev Drug Discov 2009;8(2):129–38.

82. Merkel OM, Rubinstein I, Kissel T. siRNA delivery to the lung: what's new? Adv Drug Deliv Rev 2014;75: 112–28.

83. Chen Y, Gu H, Zhang DS, et al. Highly effective inhibition of lung cancer growth and metastasis by systemic delivery of siRNA via multimodal mesoporous silica-based nanocarrier. Biomaterials 2014;35(38): 10058–69.

84. Guo C, Al-Jamal WT, Toma FM, et al. Design of cationic multiwalled carbon nanotubes as efficient siRNA vectors for lung cancer xenograft eradication. Bioconjug Chem 2015;26(7):1370–9.

85. Luk BT, Zhang L. Current advances in polymer-based nanotheranostics for cancer treatment and diagnosis. ACS Appl Mater Inter 2014;6(24): 21859–73.

86. Wang C, Ravi S, Garapati US, et al. Multifunctional chitosan magnetic-graphene (CMG) nanoparticles: a theranostic platform for tumor-targeted co- delivery of drugs, genes and MRI contrast agents. J Mater Chem B Mater Biol Med 2013;1(35): 4396–405.

87. Khullar OV, Griset AP, Gibbs-Strauss SL, et al. Nanoparticle migration and delivery of Paclitaxel to regional lymph nodes in a large animal model. J Am Coll Surg 2012;214(3):328–37.

88. Khullar O, Frangioni JV, Grinstaff M, et al. Image-guided sentinel lymph node mapping and nanotechnology-based nodal treatment in lung cancer using invisible near-infrared fluorescent light. Semin Thorac Cardiovasc Surg 2009;21(4): 309–15.

Present and Future Application of Energy Devices in Thoracic Surgery

Eric Goudie, MD[a], Mehdi Tahiri, MD[b],
Moishe Liberman, MD, PhD[c],*

KEYWORDS

- Electrosurgery • Minimally invasive surgery • Vascular sealing • Endoscopic procedures
- Radiofrequency ablation

KEY POINTS

- There is growing evidence that ultrasonic shears are effective and safe for pulmonary artery branch ligation of 7 mm diameter or less.
- Palliation of esophageal cancer with brachytherapy has been largely replaced by endoluminal stenting.
- Radiofrequency ablation is an interesting treatment option for inoperable patients, although it has been replaced by stereotactic body radiation therapy otherwise known as stereotactic ablative radiotherapy.
- Argon plasma coagulation is useful in the treatment of endobronchial lesions and for hemostasis; its tissue penetration of 2 to 3 mm makes it a relatively safe energy device.
- Cryoablation does not destroy tissue instantaneously; it can control malignant airway lesions in non–life-threatening situations and is contraindicated in life-threatening airway obstruction.

INTRODUCTION

In 1920, Dr William T. Bovie, a physicist at Harvard in collaboration with the neurosurgeon Dr Harvey W. Cushing, created the first electrosurgical unit.[1] Since the creation of this first unit, there have been important developments in the field of energy devices with the emergence of new technologies including ultrasonic devices. Today, the vast majority of surgical procedures performed involve energy devices for tissue cutting, dissection, and vessel sealing.[2] Although most surgeons use these devices in their daily practice, a majority of them are not familiar with the technology behind them, or their applications.[3]

In the last decade, there has been an incremental use of video assisted thoracoscopic surgery (VATS) for the treatment of lung disease owing to the multiple benefits of the procedure, such as decreased pain, decreased morbidity, and shorter

The authors report no commercial or financial conflicts of interest. There are no funding sources.
[a] Thoracic Surgery Laboratory, CHUM Endoscopic Tracheobronchial and Oesophageal Center (CETOC), Centre Hospitalier de l'Université de Montréal, University of Montreal, 1560 Sherbrooke Street Est, 8e CD - Pavillon Lachapelle, Suite D-8051, Montreal, Quebec H2L 4M1, Canada; [b] Thoracic Surgery Laboratory, CHUM Endoscopic Tracheobronchial and Oesophageal Center (CETOC), Centre Hospitalier de l'Université de Montréal, 1560 Sherbrooke Street Est, 8e CD - Pavillon Lachapelle, Suite D-8051, Montreal, Quebec H2L 4M1, Canada; [c] Division of Thoracic Surgery, Department of Surgery, CHUM Endoscopic Tracheobronchial and Oesophageal Center (CETOC), Centre Hospitalier de l'Université de Montréal, University of Montreal, 1560 Sherbrooke Street Est, 8e CD - Pavillon Lachapelle, Suite D-8051, Montreal, Quebec H2L 4M1, Canada
* Corresponding author.
E-mail address: moishe.liberman@umontreal.ca

duration of hospital stay.[4] However, there remains a minority of anatomic pulmonary resections that are being performed by VATS.[5] For example, in VATS lobectomy, the technical difficulty is primarily related to pulmonary artery (PA) branch manipulation and the perceived and actual danger of potentially injuring the PA while using an endostapler. This is owing to the size, rigidity, and footprint of the endostaplers devices. Energy devices have the potential to overcome these limitations, hence making these procedures safer and less stressful for the surgeon, and therefore more prevalent for anatomic pulmonary resections. They have a smaller footprint and are easier to manipulate around short and small PA branches.

In this article, we review the present and future applications of energy devices in thoracic surgery.

ELECTROCAUTERY: MONOPOLAR AND BIPOLAR DEVICES

The concept of electrosurgery refers to the use of a high-frequency electric current to cut tissue and coagulate vessels.[6] In electrosurgery, the flow of electricity requires a complete pathway that includes the electrosurgical generator (high-frequency oscillator and an amplifier) with the patient plates (inactive dispersive electrodes), the connecting cables and the active electrode.[7] The generator is the source of electron flow and voltage, it takes 60 cycles current and increase it to more than 200,000 cycles per second. At this frequency, electrosurgical energy can pass through the patient with minimal neuromuscular stimulation and no risk of electrocution. The patient tissue represents the impedance, producing heat as the electrons overcome the impedance.[8] There are 2 main types of electrocautery devices that are used in electrosurgery: monopolar and bipolar devices.

With monopolar electrosurgery, energy flows from the generator to the active electrode, and then the energy passes through the patient to the dispersive cautery pad, thus completing the electrical circuit.[9] There are 3 main monopolar modes used to produce the different tissue effect: (1) cut, (2) coag, and (3) blend.[10] Cut uses a constant waveform to vaporize (cut) the tissue. Using the coag waveform, the duty cycle is reduced. Coag waveform produces less heat and, instead of vaporization, a tissue coagulum is produced. The blend current is a modification in the duty cycle of these 2 forms.

In bipolar electrosurgery, 2 electrodes serve as the equivalent of the active and dispersive leads in the monopolar mode. The electrical current is confined to the tissue between the tines of the

bipolar forceps. The LigaSure (LS) device (Medtronic, Covidien, Boulder, CO) is a bipolar device that delivers high current at a low voltage along with the pressure from the jaw to tissue. However, this system differs from classical bipolar devices, with an incorporated technology that monitors the energy expended while denaturing the collagen and elastin within the vessel walls. During the cooling phase of the cycle, cross-linking re-occurs, creating a new seal.

A study by Lacin and associates[11] in 2007 evaluated the capacity of LigaSure in sealing of PAs. They used the LigaSure device to seal and divide the main lobar PAs and veins in 12 sheep. The sheep were divided into 2 groups. The first group underwent right lower lobectomy and were humanely killed immediately. The second group underwent right upper lobectomy in a 7-day survival model. The vascular dehiscence rate was very high in the first group (2 of 6 PAs and 3 of 6 pulmonary veins >9 mm). There was no vascular dehiscence in the second group that contained pulmonary vessels smaller than 7 mm.

Tsunezuka and colleagues[12] evaluated the bursting pressure of PAs sealed with the LigaSure device in a human model during VATS lung resection. LigaSure was used to seal segmental and subsegmental PAs less than 5 mm in diameter. PAs larger than 5 mm and smaller than 10 mm were secured with proximal ligation with a 1-0 unidentified suture followed by LigaSure sealing. PAs greater than 10 mm were divided using endostaplers. PAs sealed with LigaSure in this study achieved high bursting pressures with higher bursting pressures in PAs smaller than 5 mm compared with PAs larger than 5 mm (607 vs 447 mm Hg). Another group from Japan described the use of LigaSure in the division of intersegmental PA branches in 2 VATS segmentectomies in 2011.[13] However, once again, vessels sealed with LigaSure were secured with proximal ligation. There were no bleeding episodes.

Albanese[14] reported on 14 total energy VATS lobectomies in 3- to 15-month old children. LigaSure was used to transect the main pulmonary vessels and complete the fissure. There were no intraoperative or postoperative complications. Another series of 6 total energy VATS lobectomies in children was published in 2006. The LigaSure device was used to seal the pulmonary lobar vessels, while the bronchi were sealed with interrupted sutures. There were no intraoperative complications. Two patients had postoperative hemothorax, which resolved without a second intervention.[15]

PA ligation and sealing is a critical step in anatomic lung resection. During VATS lobectomy,

PA sealing is typically performed using endostaplers or clips. Studies assessing the capacity of LigaSure to seal PA have not shown enough evidence at this time to determine the safety of LigaSure for PA sealing. Furthermore, in a study conducted by our group, we showed that ultrasound sealing technology seems to be superior to advanced bipolar technology in sealing PA branches, and might be a more suitable device to seal PAs in vivo.[16]

ULTRASONIC DEVICES

Ultrasonic shears use both compression and friction to deliver mechanical energy to target tissue. Amino acids unwind and reshape and hydrogen bonds break, resulting in a sticky coagulum. Ultrasonic shears contain piezoelectric disks that convert electric energy into mechanical energy, which is amplified by a silicone element. Vibration generates vapor within the cells that lead to disruption and fragmentation.

The Harmonic Scalpel (Ethicon Endosurgery, Cincinnati, OH) was the first energy device assessed in pulmonary parenchymal resection (lung sealing) in 1999. The Harmonic Scalpel was used in limited lung resection in 30 consecutive patients. The lung parenchyma was resected using the Harmonic Scalpel; however, the resected lung surfaces were then oversewn with absorbable suture. There were no intraoperative episodes of bleeding.[17] In 2004, Molnar and colleagues[18] compared the Harmonic Scalpel with endostaplers in pulmonary parenchymal wedge resection (3 × 5 cm) in 8 dogs. There was no difference in results between the 2 groups in terms of air leak, bleeding, or histopathologic healing. Lungs resected with the Harmonic Scalpel showed less granulomatous formation in the resection line.[18] In 2005, the same group randomized 40 consecutive patients undergoing VATS lung biopsies (wedge resection) to 2 groups using either the Harmonic Scalpel or endostaplers. There were no intraoperative complications. Postoperative complications were similar in both groups. The operative time was less with the Harmonic Scalpel.[19] The same group reported a high rate of air leaks requiring drainage in another study analyzing a 16 patient series of Harmonic Scalpel lung resection.[20]

In 2007, Nicastri and colleagues[21] demonstrated the efficacy of the Harmonic Scalpel in dividing and sealing pulmonary vessels less than 4 mm diameter in an animal survival model. However, in the same study, complete and permanent PA sealing was achieved in only 25% of 5-mm PAs, 33% of 7-mm Pas, and 0% of 9-mm PAs.

In another study published in 2009, the Harmonic scalpel was used to seal 43 PAs and 13 pulmonary veins in animal model. The bursting pressure of the arteries sealed was more than 75 mm Hg. The same group used the Harmonic Scalpel to seal and divide pulmonary vessels 5 mm or less in diameter in 20 patients who underwent VATS anatomic lung resection. However, the sealed vessels were also secured with a single proximal ligation. PAs larger than 5 mm were divided by endostapler. There were no postoperative bleeding episodes.[22]

A study published in 2010 observed a high rate of late (1–3 months) presentation of bronchopleural fistulas in the patients having undergone Harmonic Scalpel segementectomy. The Harmonic Scalpel was used to seal the bronchial airway to the resected segment. The incidence of bronchopleural fistula was 45% in this 11-patient series. There were no intraoperative air leaks with an intraoperative bronchial underwater bubble test and all patients had an uneventful postoperative course. The histologic analysis showed that the Harmonic Scalpel sealed bronchi were reduced in size; however, the lumens were still patent.[23]

Our group recently published a study evaluating four commonly used energy sealing devices Harmonic Ace (Ethicon), Thunderbeat (Olympus, Tokyo, Japan), LigaSure (LS) (Covidien), and Enseal (Ethicon).[16] After anatomic lung resection in human subjects, the PA branches were dissected on the back table. To simulate normal PA pressure during sealing, a closed circuit of distally ligated PAs was created and the vessel was pressurized to 25 mm Hg. Sealing was then performed with one of the sealing devices, the vessel was slowly pressurized and the bursting pressure was recorded. Results showed that the Harmonic Scalpel demonstrated bursting pressures in excess of 300 mm Hg (≤822 mm Hg) in segmental and subsegmental PAs with diameters from 3 to 13 mm. On the other hand, segmental and subsegmental PAs sealed with Ligasure demonstrated bursting pressures of only 233 mm Hg for PAs of less than 5 mm in diameter and 178 mm Hg for PAs of greater than 5 mm in diameter.

Our study and the current literature suggest that ultrasound sealing technology seems to be superior to advanced bipolar technology in sealing PA branches. However, further research is needed to determine the long-term safety of PA energy sealing in an in vivo environment.

In the last few years, adaptive tissue technology has been developed to provide greater precision through improved energy delivery in ultrasonic devices. With adaptive tissue technology, unnecessary power output that could lead to thermal injury is reduced while achieving adequate hemostasis.[24] Our group conducted a study evaluating PA branch sealing with an ultrasonic energy vessel-sealing device using adaptive tissue technology in VATS lobectomy on a canine survival model. Ten adult dogs underwent VATS lobectomy. All the steps of a standard VATS lobectomy technique were followed, except for PA branch sealing. The Harmonic Ace+7 (Ethicon) was used to replace vascular endostaplers for all PA branches. Dogs were kept alive for 30 days and followed for any hemorrhagic complication.

The mean in vivo PA diameter was 5.6 mm (range, 2–12). The mean ex vivo PA diameter was 5.5 mm (range, 2–14 mm). One PA branch with a diameter of 10 mm had a partial seal failure immediately at the time of sealing. The device was reapplied on the stump and the PA branch was sealed successfully. All dogs survived for 30 days without hemothorax. Necropsy at 30 days did not reveal any signs of postoperative bleeding. Pathology of the sealed PA branches at 30 days revealed fibrosis, giant cell reaction, neovascularization, and thermal changes of the vessel wall.

The Harmonic Ace+7 was safe for PA sealing in VATS lobectomy in an animal survival model. Human studies are needed to determine safety in human VATS lobectomy. The use of ultrasonic energy vessel-sealing device on PA branches may decrease the risk of iatrogenic PA injury.

BRACHYTHERAPY

Brachytherapy (BT) is a form of local radiation treatment that involves temporary placement of encapsulated radioactive sources within or near the tumor. Endobronchial BT (EBBT) is used mainly as a palliative therapy for the treatment of non–small-cell lung cancer involving the airway.[25] It can also be used for curative intent treatment in airway tumors in the inoperable patient. In the esophagus, it is a technique that had a major role in esophageal cancer palliation of dysphagia; however, it has been largely replaced in recent years with esophageal endoluminal stenting. There are several advantages of BT in comparison to external beam radiation, including (1) a higher dose of radiation to the tumor, (2) minimization of the radiation exposure to normal tissue, and (3) precise dose location.

EBBT is performed by placing the radioactive source through a hollow catheter that is placed into the endobronchial tree under bronchoscopic guidance. The flexible bronchoscope is then removed, the position of the catheter is then confirmed by a radiograph and the catheter is loaded with iridium 192.

EBBT can be delivered either by a high dose rate or low dose rate. High dose rate EBBT is usually the common way to provide this therapy because treatment times are shorter, making it an outpatient procedure. In addition, there is less catheter displacement and treatment costs are reduced.[26]

In a metaanalysis by the Cochrane group comparing the use of EBBT with external beam radiation therapy, the authors conclude that there was no evidence to recommend EBBT over external beam radiation therapy. The results suggested also that external beam radiation therapy alone is more effective than EBBT.[27] However, there remain certain circumstances and select patient populations where BT can be useful.

RADIOFREQUENCY ABLATION

Radiofrequency energy use in thoracic surgery has been gaining interest in the past 15 years for lung tumor ablation. Nevertheless, to this day there is no randomized trial evaluating its use. Radiofrequency ablation (RFA) uses heat induced by an electrode placed in the lung tumor to induce cell death. Because surgery is the gold standard for stage I lung cancer, RFA is an interesting treatment option for inoperable patients. However, over the last few years, this technique has been largely replaced by stereotactic body radiation therapy, which is otherwise known as stereotactic ablative radiotherapy.

For RFA, a 14- to 21-G electrode is placed percutaneously inside the tumor under computed tomography (CT), MR, or ultrasound guidance. The electrode is attached to a generator and a conductive plate is installed on the patient to return the energy of this monopolar device back to the generator. The shaft of the needle is insulated leaving only the tip of the device exposed to transmit current. The generator induces radiofrequencies between 375 and 500 kHz, which is translated into an electric field around the tip of the electrode. The oscillating current of the electric field makes the ions in the tissues surrounding the electrode oscillate in the same fashion. This frictional movement within the tissue itself creates heat.[28] The temperature the tissue will reach depends on the total energy transmitted, tissue characteristics, and heat loss occurring in the tissue.[29]

The goal of this technology is to induce tumor cell death by a process called coagulation necrosis. A brief exposure to temperatures of 60°C or more are needed to cause cellular damage that will lead to cell death.[30] Temperatures under

60°C will take longer time to cause enough cellular damage. For example, prostatic tissue heated at 45°C will take 1 hour to cause cellular death.[31] Temperatures above 105°C must be avoided because temperatures this high will cause boiling, vaporization, and carbonization, thus preventing proper heat spread in the tissue. The gas produced acts as an insulation.[32] However, this property in lung parenchyma has the advantage of limiting heat spread in aerated lung parenchyma.[33]

Different RFA systems are commercially available and include monopolar electrodes, multiprobe arrays, and internally cooled electrodes. Monopolar electrodes are for small tumors usually not exceeding 1.6 cm diameter, because the minimal heat required for tissue destruction might not be reached at a wider diameter. Multiprobe arrays overcome this limitation in larger tumors by deploying multiple tips creating multiple foci inducing an electric field. Coagulation necrosis up to 5 cm diameter can be achieved.[30] Internally cooled electrodes have 2 channels to have fluid circulation to cool the tip of the electrode. Preventing the tissue surrounding the tip of the electrode to overheat permits the heat to spread further away from tip.

Several retrospective and prospective studies evaluating RFA in lung cancer have been published.[34–46] For stage I lung cancer, 2-year survival rates that vary between 50% and 93% and 5-year survival rates that vary between 35% and 40% have been reported.[34,41,44–47] Tumors larger than 3 cm in diameter are associated with a higher recurrence rate after RFA. Ambrogi and colleagues[45] published a series of 80 RFAs in 57 nonoperable patients with stage I non–small cell lung cancer. Lesion size varied from 1.1 to 5.0 cm (mean, 2.6). All procedures were technically successful and no procedure-related mortality was recorded. Four cases of pneumothorax requiring drainage were reported. The cancer-specific survival rates at 1, 3, and 5 years were 89%, 59%, and 40%, respectively. Lanuti and colleagues[41] reported 2- and 4-year survival rates of 78% and 47% in 31 stage I lung cancer patients considered ineligible for resection. Complications included pneumothorax requiring chest tube insertion (8%), minor hemoptysis (16%), hemothorax (5%), pneumonia (16%), pleural effusion (21%) right recurrent laryngeal nerve palsy (1 case), and bronchopleural fistula (8%). There was no 30-day mortality.

One of the largest series evaluating complications reported a 0.4% mortality rate in 1000 RFA sessions in 420 patients with 1403 lung tumors.[48] Causes of death were interstitial pneumonia (n = 3) and hemothorax (n = 1). The major complication rate was 9.8% (pleurisy, pneumonia, lung abscess, bleeding, pneumothorax, bronchopleural fistula, nerve injury). One case of diaphragm injury and 1 case of tumor seeding were reported.

One of the limitations of this technique is the assessment of the zone that needs to be treated. Most lung RFAs are done under CT scan guidance. Immediately after RFA treatment, ground-glass lesions appear on CT scan. According to animal studies, a minimal safety margin of 4.1 mm must be obtained to include the tissue needing to be ablated.[49,50] The peripheral margins seen on CT scan may contain viable cells. However, even with safety margins, there is no way to confirm that all tumor tissue has been ablated. Another challenge associated with RFA is follow-up. Combined chest CT and PET imaging are part of an adequate follow-up strategy; however, it is very difficult to assess success of treatment or early local recurrence using these techniques.[51]

ARGON PLASMA COAGULATION

Argon plasma coagulation (APC) has gained interest in the past years for the treatment of endobronchial lesions and for hemostasis. Most of its application is in the palliative context, but it is also one of the therapeutic options in the management of airway bleeding and the treatment of benign lesions. APC has an immediate effect on tissue in comparison with other endobronchial energy devices such as cryoablation and BT. APC is useful in the chest or abdominal cavity for diffuse bleeding and is specifically useful in the treatment of diffuse bleeding from the chest wall after extrapleural resection or dissection.

APC is a type of electrocautery device that requires specific equipment. A probe is attached to a generator and an argon gas cylinder. A conductive plate is attached to the patient to return the current to the generator. Argon gas is released at the tip of the probe and a high voltage current is generated. The argon gas then becomes ionized and a monopolar current reaches the tissue surrounding the argon gas.[52] The effect penetrates 2 to 3 mm deep in the tissue. This property of APC makes it an interesting energy source because its low penetration reduces risks of airway perforation.

APC best treats endoluminal lesions in the central airway, but can also reach lesions in lobar and segmental bronchi. APC cannot treat airway obstruction owing to extrinsic compression. In a study of 372 patients in whom APC was performed 482 times, success was obtained in 124 of 186 patients with airway obstruction.[53] Another study reporting 39 patients with obstructing lesions showed improvement in symptoms in 38 patients after treatment with APC.[54] Endobronchial lesions that are best treated with APC are less than 4 cm, superficial, flat, or polypoid and located at the bifurcation of the airway. Because it immediately destroys tissue, APC can be useful in life-threatening airway obstructions.

Benign lesions are also amenable to treatment with APC. These include benign strictures from granulation tissue, benign polyp removal, and Dieulafoy disease. Successful endobronchial abscess drainage also has been reported.[55]

APC is part of the treatment strategy in airway bleeding from malignant and benign lesions. Reichle and colleagues[53] reported bleeding control in 118 of 119 patients presenting with hemoptysis. Similar results were reported by Morice and colleagues[54] in achieving hemostasis in all 56 patients treated in their series.

Added to standard contraindications to bronchoscopic procedures, contraindications to endobronchial APC include high flow oxygen (FiO_2 >40%), airway obstruction occurring only from extrinsic airway obstruction, and absence of viable lung tissue distal to the lesion and possibility of curative treatment.

Complications from endobronchial APC range from 0.5% to 4%. Airway burns or fire are rare and strategies can be used to reduce the risk. These include using minimal FiO_2 (<40%), limiting the power set on the probe <80 watts, and limiting the application time of the probe to less than 3 seconds. Other reported complications are airway perforation, hemorrhage, and gas embolism.

CRYOTHERAPY/CRYOABLATION

Cryoablation freezes tissue using either nitrous oxide or liquid nitrogen. Repeated rapid cooling of tissue under 20°C results in cell death by causing intracellular ice crystal formation.[56] Another mechanism of cell destruction results from ischemic necrosis as the microcirculation around the tissue significantly reduces blood flow from the freezing effects on microcirculation. Hence, cryoablation does not instantaneously destroy tissue, it takes days to week to reach full effect. The effect of cryoablation penetrates approximately 3 mm into the tissue.[57]

Cryoablation can achieve control of malignant airway lesions in non–life-threatening situations. Schumann published a series of 225 patients who underwent cryoablation for malignant airway stenosis.[58] The procedure was successful in 205 patients (91.1%). Ten patients required a combination with a second endobronchial technique to achieve control. Cryoablation has been suggested as a possible curative treatment strategy for typical carcinoid tumors, however it is this has not been validated in prospective controlled trials and is not considered standard of care for operable patients.[59]

Cryoablation is less recognized as a treatment option for benign airway lesions. Reported lesions treated with cryoablation include granulation tissue, endobronchial lipomas, hamartomas and hemangiomas. Caution must be used not to apply cryoablation on fibrotic tissue as it can cause further stenosis.

Complications include mucus plugging from tissue shedding in the days and weeks after the treatment. A repeat bronchoscopy is sometimes needed to clean the debris. Other complications are similar to other endobronchial ablation techniques and include hemorrhage and airway perforation.

SUMMARY

In the last decade, many energy devices have entered day-to-day practice in thoracic surgery. Some have proven and recognized applications, as others still require further trials. Nevertheless, currently used devices continue to be improved upon and new applications for current devices will be evaluated. Ultimately, novel applications of energy in thoracic surgery and refinement in technology will hopefully allow for safer and less invasive techniques for patients requiring thoracic surgical procedures.

REFERENCES

1. O'Connor JL, Bloom DA, William T. Bovie and electrosurgery. Surgery 1996;119(4):390–6.
2. Madani A, Watanabe Y, Vassiliou MC, et al. Impact of a hands-on component on learning in the Fundamental Use of Surgical Energy (FUSE) curriculum: a randomized-controlled trial in surgical trainees. Surg Endosc 2014;28(10):2772–82.
3. Feldman LS, Fuchshuber P, Jones DB, et al. Surgeons don't know what they don't know about the safe use of energy in surgery. Surg Endosc 2012;26(10):2735–9.
4. Scott WJ, Allen MS, Darling G, et al. Video-assisted thoracic surgery versus open lobectomy for lung cancer: a secondary analysis of data from the American College of Surgeons Oncology Group Z0030 randomized clinical trial. J Thorac Cardiovasc Surg 2010;139(4):976–81 [discussion: 81–3].
5. Paul S, Sedrakyan A, Chiu YL, et al. Outcomes after lobectomy using thoracoscopy vs thoracotomy: a

comparative effectiveness analysis utilizing the nationwide inpatient sample database. Eur J Cardiothorac Surg 2013;43(4):813–7.

6. Taheri A, Mansoori P, Sandoval LF, et al. Electrosurgery: part I. Basics and principles. J Am Acad Dermatol 2014;70(4):591.e1–14 [quiz: 605–6].

7. Vilos GA, Rajakumar C. Electrosurgical generators and monopolar and bipolar electrosurgery. J Minim Invasive Gynecol 2013;20(3):279–87.

8. Alkatout I, Schollmeyer T, Hawaldar NA, et al. Principles and safety measures of electrosurgery in laparoscopy. JSLS 2012;16(1):130–9

9. Odell RC. Surgical complications specific to monopolar electrosurgical energy: engineering changes that have made electrosurgery safer. J Minim Invasive Gynecol 2013;20(3):288–98.

10. Fyock CJ, Draganov PV. Colonoscopic polypectomy and associated techniques. World J Gastroenterol 2010;16(29):3630–7.

11. Lacin T, Batirel HF, Ozer K, et al. Safety of a thermal vessel sealer on main pulmonary vessels. Eur J Cardiothorac Surg 2007;31(3):482–5 [discussion: 485].

12. Tsunezuka Y, Waseda R, Yachi T. Electrothermal bipolar vessel sealing device LigaSureV for pulmonary artery ligation–burst pressure and clinical experiences in complete video-assisted thoracoscopic major lung resection for lung cancer. Interact Cardiovasc Thorac Surg 2010;11(3):229–33.

13. Watanabe A, Miyajima M, Kawaharada N, et al. Two separate thoroscopic segmentectomies with vessel sealing system. Eur J Cardiothorac Surg 2012; 41(4):e62–4.

14. Albanese CT, Sydorak RM, Tsao K, et al. Thoracoscopic Lobectomy for Prenatally Diagnosed Lung Lesions. J Pediatr Surg 2003;38:553–5.

15. Cano I, Anton-Pacheco JL, García A, et al. Video-assisted thoracoscopic lobectomy in infants. Eur J Cardiothorac Surg 2006;29(6):997–1000.

16. Liberman M, Khereba M, Goudie E, et al. Pilot study of pulmonary arterial branch sealing using energy devices in an ex vivo model. J Thorac Cardiovasc Surg 2014;148(6):3219–23.

17. Aoki T, Kaseda S. Thoracoscopic resection of the lung with the ultrasonic scalpel. Ann Thorac Surg 1999;67(4):1181–3.

18. Molnar TF, Szanto Z, Laszlo T, et al. Cutting lung parenchyma using the harmonic scalpel–an animal experiment. Eur J Cardiothorac Surg 2004;26(6): 1192–5.

19. Molnar TF, Benko I, Szanto Z, et al. Lung biopsy using harmonic scalpel: a randomised single institute study. Eur J Cardiothorac Surg 2005;28(4): 604–6.

20. Molnar TF, Benko I, Szanto Z, et al. Complications after ultrasonic lung parenchyma biopsy: a strong note for caution. Surg Endosc 2008;22(3):679–82.

21. Nicastri DG, Wu M, Yun J, et al. Evaluation of efficacy of an ultrasonic scalpel for pulmonary vascular ligation in an animal model. J Thorac Cardiovasc Surg 2007;134(1):160–4.

22. Tanaka T, Ueda K, Hayashi M, et al. Clinical application of an ultrasonic scalpel to divide pulmonary vessels based on laboratory evidence. Interact Cardiovasc Thorac Surg 2009;8(6):615–8.

23. Takagi K, Hata Y, Sasamoto S, et al. Late onset postoperative pulmonary fistula following a pulmonary segmentectomy using electrocautery or a harmonic scalpel. Ann Thorac Cardiovasc Surg 2010;16(1): 21–5.

24. Broughton D, Welling AL, Monroe EH, et al. Tissue effects in vessel sealing and transection from an ultrasonic device with more intelligent control of energy delivery. Med Devices (Auckl) 2013;6: 151–4.

25. Hennequin C, Bleichner O, Tredaniel J, et al. Endobronchial brachytherapy: technique and indications. Cancer Radiother 2003;7(1):33–41 [in French].

26. Celebioglu B, Gurkan OU, Erdogan S, et al. High dose rate endobronchial brachytherapy effectively palliates symptoms due to inoperable lung cancer. Jpn J Clin Oncol 2002;32(11):443–8.

27. Reveiz L, Rueda JR, Cardona AF. Palliative endobronchial brachytherapy for non-small cell lung cancer. Cochrane Database Syst Rev 2012;(12):CD004284.

28. Organ LW. Electrophysiologic principles of radiofrequency lesion making. Appl Neurophysiol 1976; 39(2):69–76.

29. Pennes HH. Analysis of tissue and arterial blood temperatures in the resting human forearm. J Appl Physiol 1948;1(2):93–122.

30. Goldberg SN, Dupuy DE. Image-guided radiofrequency tumor ablation: challenges and opportunities—Part I. J Vasc Interv Radiol 2001;12(9): 1021–32.

31. Larson TR, Bostwick DG, Corica A. Temperature-correlated histopathologic changes following microwave thermoablation of obstructive tissue in patients with benign prostatic hyperplasia. Urology 1996; 47(4):463–9.

32. Goldberg SN, Gazelle GS, Mueller PR. Thermal ablation therapy for focal malignancy: a unified approach to underlying principles, techniques, and diagnostic imaging guidance. AJR Am J Roentgenol 2000;174(2):323–31.

33. Goldberg SN, Gazelle GS, Compton CC, et al. Radiofrequency tissue ablation in the rabbit lung: efficacy and complications. Acad Radiol 1995;2(9): 776–84.

34. Ambrogi MC, Fanucchi O, Dini P, et al. Wedge resection and radiofrequency ablation for stage I nonsmall cell lung cancer. Eur Respir J 2015;45(4): 1089–97.

35. Fernando HC, De Hoyos A, Landreneau RJ, et al. Radiofrequency ablation for the treatment of non-small cell lung cancer in marginal surgical candidates. J Thorac Cardiovasc Surg 2005;129(3): 639–44.

36. Grieco CA, Simon CJ, Mayo-Smith WW, et al. Percutaneous image-guided thermal ablation and radiation therapy: outcomes of combined treatment for 41 patients with inoperable stage I/II non-small-cell lung cancer. J Vasc Interv Radiol 2006; 17(7):1117–24.

37. Sano Y, Kanazawa S, Gobara H, et al. Feasibility of percutaneous radiofrequency ablation for intrathoracic malignancies: a large single-center experience. Cancer 2007;109(7):1397–405.

38. Choe YH, Kim SR, Lee KS, et al. The use of PTC and RFA as treatment alternatives with low procedural morbidity in non-small cell lung cancer. Eur J Cancer 2009;45(10):1773–9.

39. Pennathur A, Luketich JD, Abbas G, et al. Radiofrequency ablation for the treatment of stage I non-small cell lung cancer in high-risk patients. J Thorac Cardiovasc Surg 2007;134(4):857–64.

40. Kim SR, Han HJ, Park SJ, et al. Comparison between surgery and radiofrequency ablation for stage I non-small cell lung cancer. Eur J Radiol 2012;81(2):395–9.

41. Lanuti M, Sharma A, Digumarthy SR, et al. Radiofrequency ablation for treatment of medically inoperable stage I non-small cell lung cancer. J Thorac Cardiovasc Surg 2009;137(1):160–6.

42. Beland MD, Wasser EJ, Mayo-Smith WW, et al. Primary non-small cell lung cancer: review of frequency, location, and time of recurrence after radiofrequency ablation. Radiology 2010;254(1):301–7.

43. Simon CJ, Dupuy DE, DiPetrillo TA, et al. Pulmonary radiofrequency ablation: long-term safety and efficacy in 153 patients. Radiology 2007;243(1): 268–75.

44. Hiraki T, Gobara H, Iishi T, et al. Percutaneous radiofrequency ablation for clinical stage I non-small cell lung cancer: results in 20 nonsurgical candidates. J Thorac Cardiovasc Surg 2007;134(5):1306–12.

45. Ambrogi MC, Fanucchi O, Cioni R, et al. Long-term results of radiofrequency ablation treatment of stage I non-small cell lung cancer: a prospective intention-to-treat study. J Thorac Oncol 2011;6(12):2044–51.

46. Dupuy DE, DiPetrillo T, Gandhi S, et al. Radiofrequency ablation followed by conventional radiotherapy for medically inoperable stage I non-small cell lung cancer. Chest 2006;129(3):738–45.

47. Lencioni R, Crocetti L, Cioni R, et al. Response to radiofrequency ablation of pulmonary tumours: a prospective, intention-to-treat, multicentre clinical trial (the RAPTURE study). Lancet Oncol 2008;9(7): 621–8.

48. Kashima M, Yamakado K, Takaki H, et al. Complications after 1000 lung radiofrequency ablation sessions in 420 patients: a single center's experiences. AJR Am J Roentgenol 2011;197(4):W576–80.

49. Yamamoto A, Nakamura K, Matsuoka T, et al. Radiofrequency ablation in a porcine lung model: correlation between CT and histopathologic findings. AJR Am J Roentgenol 2005;185(5):1299–306.

50. Tominaga J, Miyachi H, Takase K, et al. Time-related changes in computed tomographic appearance and pathologic findings after radiofrequency ablation of the rabbit lung: preliminary experimental study. J Vasc Interv Radiol 2005;16(12):1719–26.

51. Abtin FG, Eradat J, Gutierrez AJ, et al. Radiofrequency ablation of lung tumors: imaging features of the postablation zone. Radiographics 2012; 32(4):947–69.

52. Platt RC. Argon plasma electrosurgical coagulation. Biomed Sci Instrum 1997;34:332–7.

53. Reichle G, Freitag L, Kullmann HJ, et al. Argon plasma coagulation in bronchology: a new method–alternative or complementary? Pneumologie 2000;54(11): 508–16 [in German].

54. Morice RC, Ece T, Ece F, et al. Endobronchial argon plasma coagulation for treatment of hemoptysis and neoplastic airway obstruction. Chest 2001;119(3): 781–7.

55. Goudie E, Kazakov J, Poirier C, et al. Endoscopic lung abscess drainage with argon plasma coagulation. J Thorac Cardiovasc Surg 2013;146(4):e35–7.

56. Gage AA, Guest K, Montes M, et al. Effect of varying freezing and thawing rates in experimental cryosurgery. Cryobiology 1985;22(2):175–82.

57. Vergnon JM, Huber RM, Moghissi K. Place of cryotherapy, brachytherapy and photodynamic therapy in therapeutic bronchoscopy of lung cancers. Eur Respir J 2006;28(1):200–18.

58. Schumann C, Hetzel M, Babiak AJ, et al. Endobronchial tumor debulking with a flexible cryoprobe for immediate treatment of malignant stenosis. J Thorac Cardiovasc Surg 2010;139(4):997–1000.

59. Bertoletti L, Elleuch R, Kaczmarek D, et al. Bronchoscopic cryotherapy treatment of isolated endoluminal typical carcinoid tumor. Chest 2006;130(5): 1405–11.

Index

http://dx.doi.org/10.1016/S1547-4127(16)00010-4
1547-4127/16/$ – see front matter © 2016 Elsevier Inc. All rights reserved.

thoracic.theclinics.com

Moving?

Make sure your subscription moves with you!

To notify us of your new address, find your **Clinics Account Number** (located on your mailing label above your name), and contact customer service at:

Email: journalscustomerservice-usa@elsevier.com

800-654-2452 (subscribers in the U.S. & Canada)
314-447-8871 (subscribers outside of the U.S. & Canada)

Fax number: 314-447-8029

Elsevier Health Sciences Division
Subscription Customer Service
3251 Riverport Lane
Maryland Heights, MO 63043

*To ensure uninterrupted delivery of your subscription, please notify us at least 4 weeks in advance of move.

Printed and bound by CPI Group (UK) Ltd, Croydon, CR0 4YY

08/05/2025

01864684-0005